SUPERCHARGED FOOD

EAT YOURSELF
BEAUTIFUL

In memory of Arthur and Paul

SUPERCHARGED FOOD

EAT YOURSELF
BEAUTIFUL

LEE HOLMES

MURDOCH BOOKS

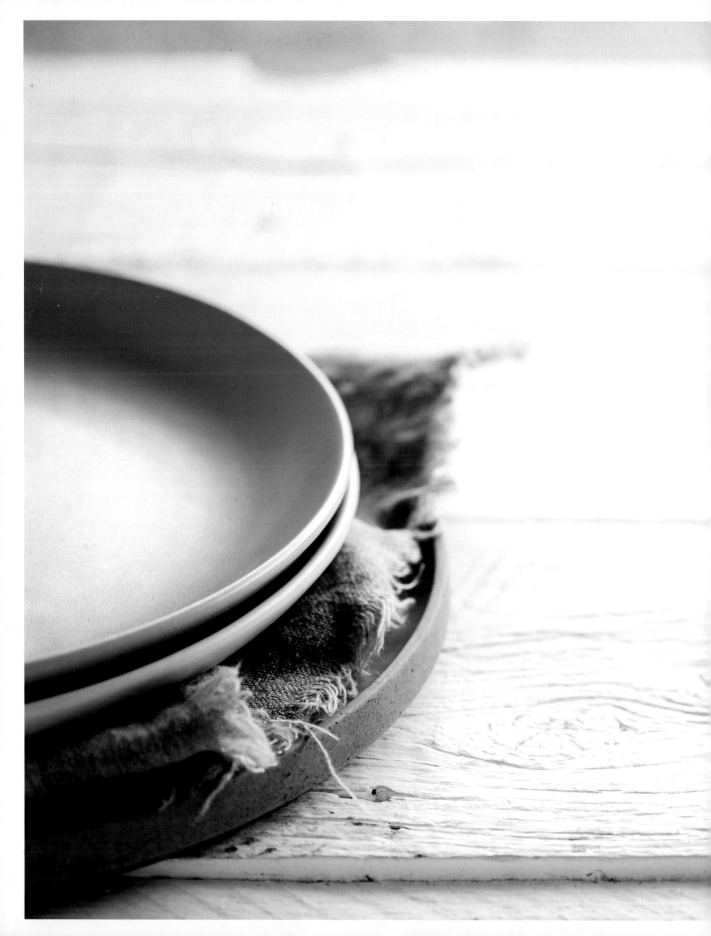

CONTENTS

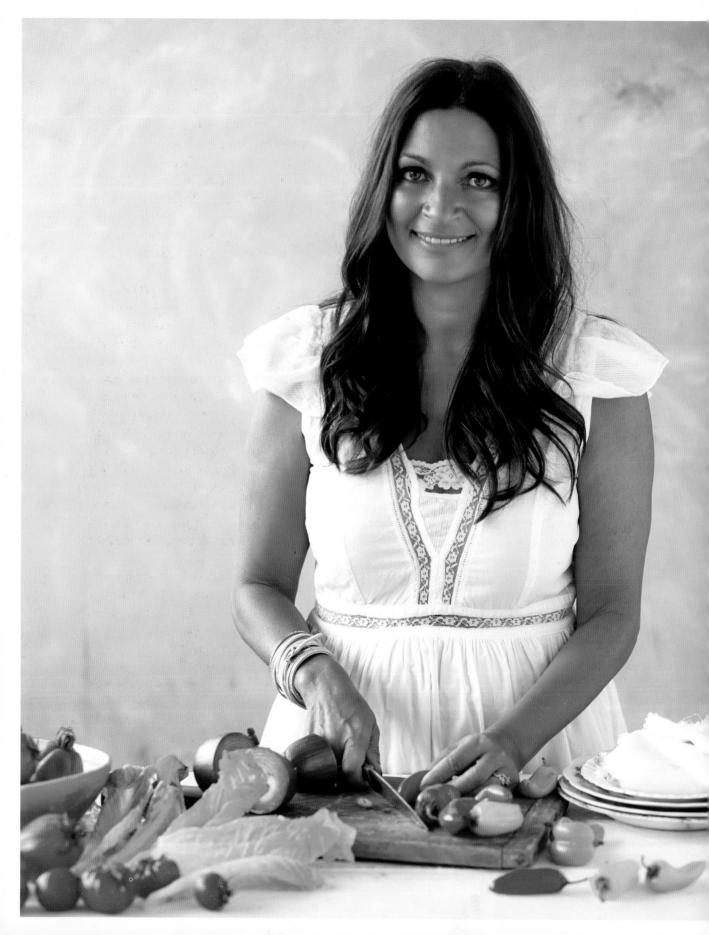

HOW TO GET STARTED

We all want to look, and feel, our very best. In our quest to do so, we often fall prey to the claims of beauty experts, inviting us to 'try this' and 'smooth that' with various creams and treatments. This book is my antidote to those beauty myths, inspired by what I have learnt in recent years on my own journey.

In 2006 I was diagnosed with fibromyalgia and all of the views I previously held on what constitutes beauty went out the window. Barely able to get out of bed in the mornings, with my hair falling out and hives covering my body, I set out on a quest to heal myself through my diet. I succeeded and in doing so I discovered that beauty – ageless, radiant, ethereal beauty – is affected more by what we feed our bodies and how we feel inside than any cream we put on our skin. I encourage you to spend your time and money at your local grocery store or farmers' market, rather than the cosmetic counter, for real foods to establish a naturally beautiful you. An authentic you.

You don't have to pay squillions of dollars for a daily supply of collagen drinks to have beautiful skin and look ageless. An inexpensive bunch of organic spinach is packed with enough collagen to boost new skin cells, plump up lips, keep skin firm and provide lustrous shiny hair, bright eyes and strong nails. Coconut fans rejoice – a coconut water will set you back just a few dollars, but will eliminate toxins and provide you with all the vital minerals required to rehydrate the skin, revealing a plumper, more hydrated complexion.

Spinach and coconut water – they're a lot cheaper than a cosmetic surgeon.

My grandmother, who believes the kitchen is the heart of the home, is still kicking on at the ripe old age of 102. She's as fit as a fiddle and her giant stack of weathered, hand-written recipes and accompanying eating principles can only be described as humble, simple and unmodified. Grandma eats a balanced diet of natural, untainted foods, limits packaged foods and says that the key to a long life is following your passions, enjoying what you do and having fun along the way.

Just as it's important to know what foods to add to your shopping cart for head-turning, truly vibrant and glowing beauty, it's also important to know your body type and love it, regardless of whether it conforms to what this month's issue of a fashion magazine tells us is beautiful. The key to aging gracefully is to accept and embrace change. A healthy mindset, along with healthy eating habits, will be reflected in a beautiful face and body.

As well as identifying and rejecting unhealthy mindsets, identifying unhealthy eating habits may keep you from nose-diving from a diet to a splurge and back again. Remember that fad diets don't work and the philosophy behind them could be hurting you more than you realise. Denying ourselves food often means that the forbidden food becomes our focus. Enter cravings.

Giving in to food cravings is a very common occurrence. Many of us spend our lives skipping from one diet to another, taking up a fad rigorously for a short period of time before giving in to our cravings and starting on the next food fad.

Have you ever told yourself, 'When my skin clears up / I lose weight / I get fit… I'll be happy'? This mindset leaves us feeling more frustrated, insecure and unhappy. The most important thing is to set yourself good intentions around how comfortable you feel with *you*. Instead of focusing on what you don't want to be, focus on how to be the best you. You'll discover that you will slowly start to have a shift in energy. This could perhaps lead you to go for a walk or take a meditation class. Take a step in a new direction and see where it leads you. With this 'new you' mindset, find a quiet space and give yourself some time to explore this book. Use the icons to discover which recipes are free from specific ingredients and best suited to your individual dietary requirements. Remember that this is not a strict diet book, but if ingredients cause you problems and create inflammation, it makes sense to avoid them.

Inflammation is the immune system's self-protection mechanism. It aims to remove harmful stimuli, including damaged cells and irritants, from the body. It is initially beneficial, but prolonged inflammation causes a raft of problems and is one of the precursors to aging and disease.

Before we get started on the recipes, you'll find some fool-proof ways to detox your skin and you'll learn about the best nutrients, vitamins, minerals and good fats to consume for a beautiful you. If you're suffering with a specific beauty condition, find out about how to rectify it with food. There's a shopping list and a meal planner to guide you once you've decided on which recipes you'd like to include. If a certain ingredient in a recipe doesn't agree with you, just swap it out for one that works for you. Remember, the recipes are just a guide for you to create the food that you enjoy eating and that make you feel beautiful.

THE KEY TO AGELESS BEAUTY

Ensuring that your body is supplied with the vitamins, minerals, amino acids and phytonutrients it needs to build your cells, improve your organs and skin's structure and reduce oxidative stress and inflammation is one of the first steps to achieve ageless beauty. Unless you have a healthy body and a clear mind, you're not going to feel beautiful.

There are many factors that can drive aging and its effects on our bodies: environmental pollution, cigarette smoke, food and cell division and degeneration. Our cells secrete inflammatory cytokines which can produce low levels of inflammation throughout the body's cells and tissues, thereby increasing the visible signs of aging.

Chronic stress is another contributor to inflammation. Stress causes the release of the hormone cortisol, which destroys brain cells, demolishes your immune system and damages your organs. Finding ways to deal with stress on a day-to-day level is imperative for your physical and mental health. Getting enough sleep at night can help you to manage your stress levels, as will engaging in a morning routine that includes gentle exercise, such as walking, stretching or yoga. These exercises jump-start the brain to release euphoric neurotransmitters. Other calming ways to start the day include meditation, writing a diary or listening to your favourite music. These methods will alleviate tension and clear your mind, readying you for the stresses of the day ahead.

It's not about being Peter Pan and looking for eternal youth. That's never going to happen. The key to aging gracefully and beautifully is to find ways to lower inflammation in the body, throw fad diets out for good and adopt a healthy way of eating following the 80/20 rule, eating well 80% of the time and giving yourself some wriggle room, indulging yourself 20% of the time. Combine that with a positive mindset and attitude to life, a sprinkling of spirituality and you have all the ingredients to enjoy life and be able to cope with its inevitable ups and downs.

The silver lining? You get to experiment in the kitchen with new ingredients and find creative ways to nourish yourself and your family.

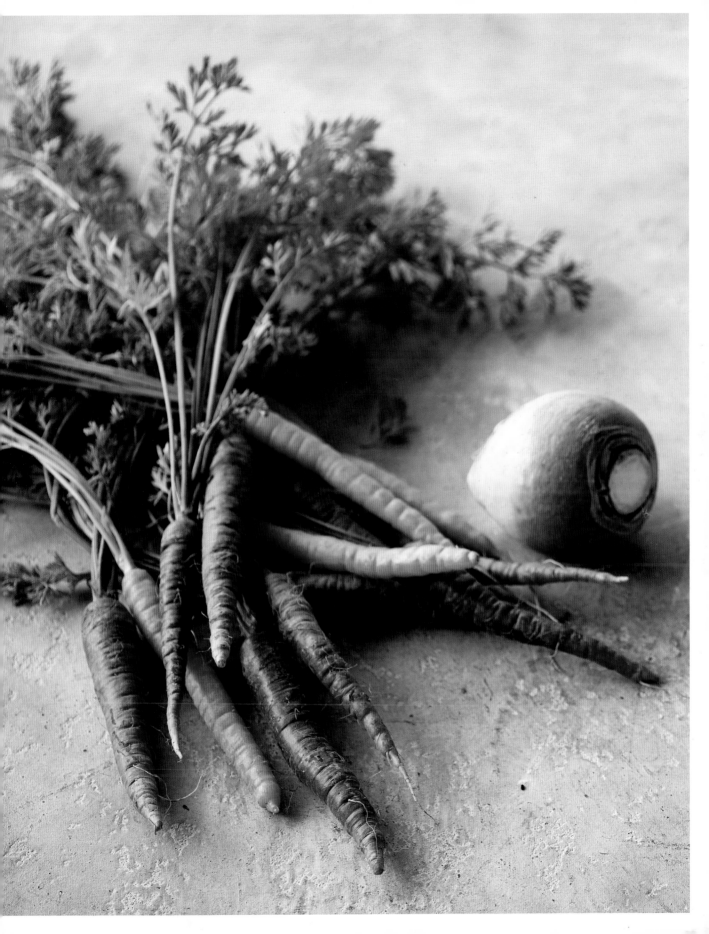

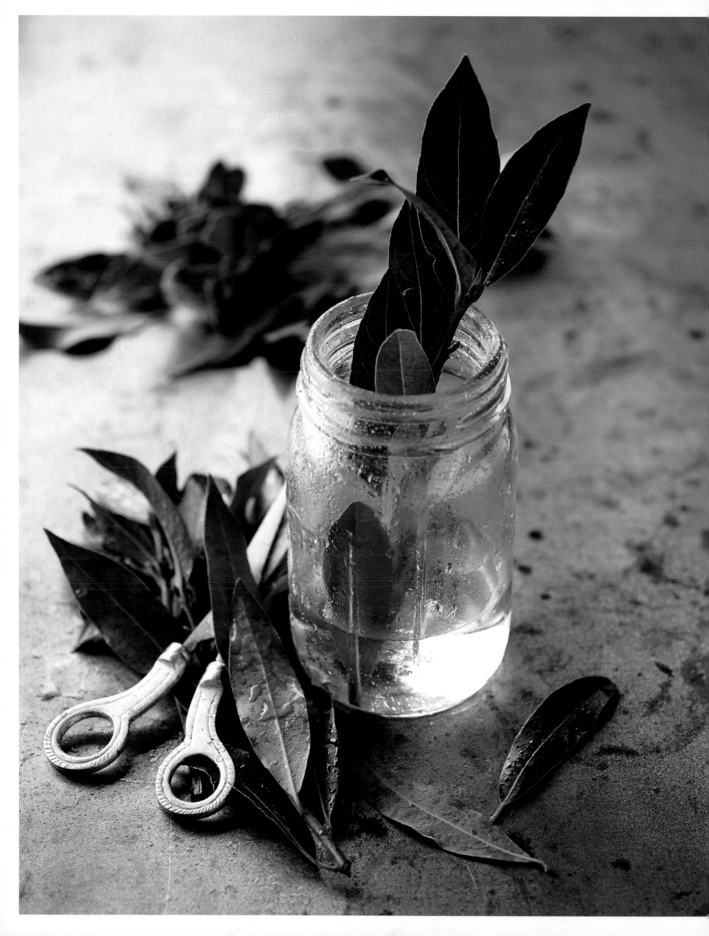

WHAT TO AVOID FOR A BEAUTIFUL YOU

Have you ever noticed how some people seem relatively unaffected by the aging process? That's because many of them are aware of how eating certain foods can accelerate aging and contribute to long-term health problems. If you're constantly making unhealthy choices when it comes to food and lifestyle, it'll have a deteriorating effect on your body and health. The average life expectancy in Australia is 79 for males and 84 for females. If you smoke over 20 cigarettes a day you can deduct three years; drink heavily, deduct seven years; if you exercise three times a week for half an hour you can add two; have a healthy diet you can add three.

Cutting out the following foods, drinks, products and supplements will not only optimise your health but also promote longevity, adding extra years to your life.

ALCOHOL: There's growing evidence that long-term or chronic alcohol consumption can cause premature and exaggerated aging to your whole body, including your brain. Alcohol activates glucocorticoid secretion which leads to elevated stress hormones circulating through the body. Chronic exposure to these hormones results in acceleration of the aging process and nerve cell degeneration. Even if you just have one glass of wine, drinking alcohol is a major dehydrator for the skin and, after a night of drinking, the effects are written all over your face. Drinking causes facial blood vessels to dilate and results in red, spidery veins across the skin. If you do drink alcohol, it's wise to drink moderately and always back up an alcoholic drink with a big glass of filtered water to minimise its adverse effects.

CAFFEINE: Caffeine temporarily boosts your level of the stress hormone cortisol, which is a stress hormone, and we all know how stress can wreak havoc on our lives. But did you know it can also accelerate aging? Your daily cup of coffee is like a wrecking ball on your skin, and if you suffer from acne or are prone to pimples, drinking coffee can exacerbate skin troubles. Due to its high temperature, coffee can also aggravate the skin by causing rosacea or redness. Caffeine acts as a diuretic, dehydrating your skin. Why not try a cup of dandelion tea every other day in place of your usual coffee? You will see the results of less anxiety and clearer skin in just a couple of weeks. Your body will thank you.

REFINED SUGARS: Consuming refined sugars can result in damaged proteins, including collagen and elastin, within your body. These protein fibres that keep your skin firm and elastic. Nowadays sugar is everywhere and pretty much anything that is labelled 'fat-free' or 'low-fat' is loaded with sugar. You'll find sugar in breakfast cereals, bread, drinks and just about all processed foods. For some alternatives to replace sugar in your recipes, flick over to pages 12–16, Alternative Sweeteners.

SOFT DRINKS: If you want to shave years off your life, soft drinks are just the ticket. But if, on the other hand, you prefer to be kind to your body and skin and remain healthy both inside and out, soft drinks need to pack their bags and get on the next coach to nowheresville. Their high sugar content can cause rapid aging and create mayhem on your blood sugar levels. And out of whack blood sugar levels can result in skin breakouts and, again, reduce your skin's natural elasticity. Aside from other unscrupulous characters such as salt, artificial sweeteners, food colourings and chemicals, soft drinks also include phosphates. Give them the flick and reap the benefits.

▰SUPERCHARGED TIP▰

The high phosphate levels in soft drinks can increase the prevalence and severity of age-related complications, such as chronic kidney disease, cardiovascular calcification, and also induce severe muscle and skin atrophy.

FRIED AND FAST FOODS: Fried and fast foods are a fast track to bad health and crepey skin. They're loaded with bad fats and often high in salt and sugar – three no-nos for maintaining your health. Their lack of nutrition is not only starving your body of healthy vitamins, but also filling it with harmful toxins. Skin breakouts will lessen by cutting out fast or fried foods and replacing them with healthy, nutrient-dense foods that are good for you, such as omega-3-rich fish, meats from grass-fed animals, lentils, healthy fats and vegetables.

CHEMICALS, TOXINS AND POLLUTANTS: We are exposed to chemicals on a daily basis. They are in most things, from the food we eat to the products we use to clean our homes and maintain our gardens. If you can avoid them, it's best to steer clear of toxic household cleaners and sprays, soaps, washing detergents, air fresheners, pesticides, insecticides and personal hygiene products, and try and replace them with non-toxic alternatives. Simple changes in your everyday routine can reduce your long-term exposure to harmful substances, such as selecting plant-based and natural varieties of products and using pump sprays instead of aerosols. Just changing the products you buy for your home to non-toxic versions will make you and your environment cleaner and will also save you money in the long-term.

PHARMACEUTICAL DRUGS: When you're exposed to pharmaceutical drugs, you're subjecting yourself to a wide range of long-term health effects and a host of side effects, some known and some unknown. We as a society are consuming more drugs for symptomatic relief than ever, but as a planet we are getting sicker. The rate of disease is on the rise. Long-term exposure to pharmaceutical drugs can have a long-term, adverse effect upon your health.

Infectious diseases are on the rise. We are becoming increasingly resistant to antibiotics and more prone to infections through dietary deficiencies. This means that we are hosting a wide variety of bacteria and viruses. When our immune systems are compromised, we are especially vulnerable to these viruses.

Research has shown that when we are deficient in antioxidants, we are unable to fight previously harmless viruses. Relying on synthetic pharmaceutical drugs for ongoing relief for non-life-threatening conditions will only increase our risk of further disease in the long-term. If you reach for a script of antibiotics, you will often end up wiping out your healthy gut bacteria. If possible, try to use a natural alternative, such as garlic – it'll be more beneficial for you in the long run. And prevention, of course, is always better than cure.

Reversing the current cycle of using drugs to cure and abate our ills, and instead looking at our nutritional profiles and eating a nutrient-rich wholefoods diet, is a key factor in warding off disease and protecting our bodies from incoming infectious diseases. That being said, you should always consult your doctor or trusted medical practitioner before adjusting your medication.

ALTERNATIVE SWEETENERS

If you want to turn back the hands of time, cutting down or eliminating sugar completely from your diet will be one of the best decisions you ever make. Sugar actively ages you by speeding up the degradation of elastin and collagen, two key skin proteins. Normalising your levels of insulin and leptin, two of the most fundamental hormones, is one of the key drivers to longevity. Consuming sugar decreases receptor sensitivity for these hormones and can lead to premature aging and age-related chronic degenerative diseases, such as diabetes and heart disease.

Cutting down on sugar, fructose, low-quality carbohydrate foods (such as pies, biscuits and sweets), and complex carbohydrates (such as bread and pasta) is a crucial step to slowing down the aging process. On the following pages are some safe sugar alternatives.

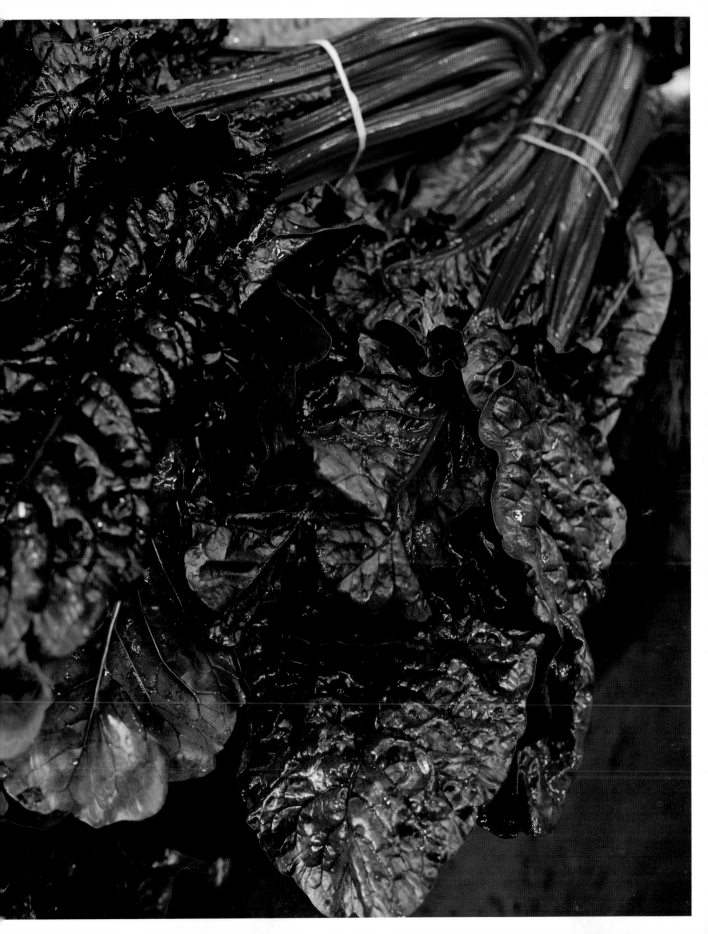

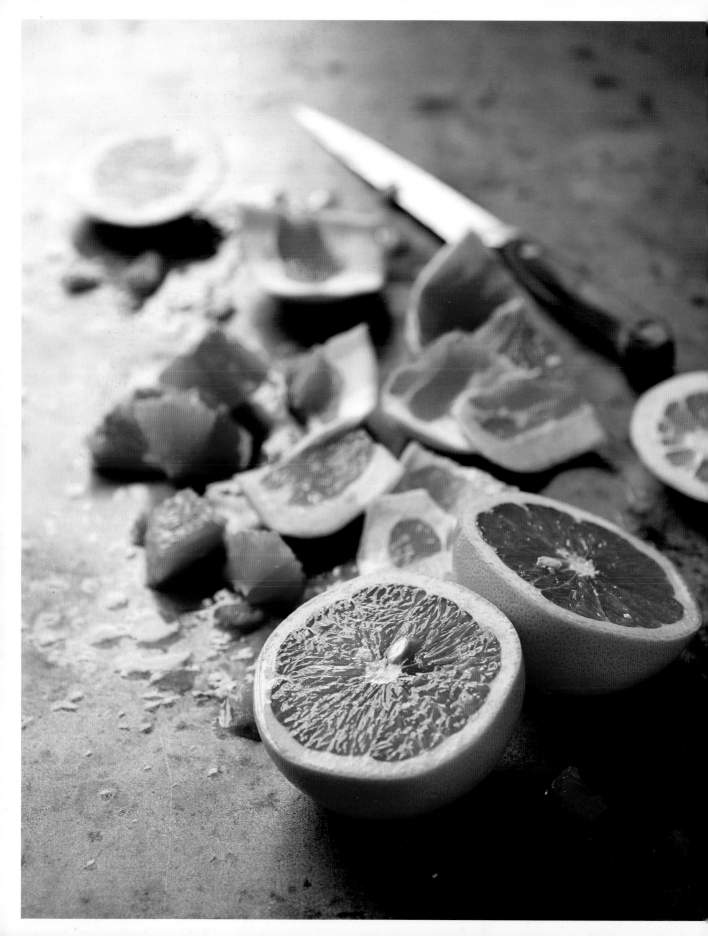

Just a word of advice: the following substitutes *can* spark sugar cravings. You'll read conflicting reports on which sugar alternative is the most virtuous – the best thing to do is find one that works for your taste buds and use it in the recipes. Remember that you can also use real fruit as a sweetener, but not if you are eliminating sugar completely from your diet.

▶SUPERCHARGED TIP◀

A quick way of identifying sugars is looking at the last letters: Anything ending in 'ose' is a sugar and anything ending in 'ol' is a sugar alcohol. Dextrins, syrups and juice concentrates are also forms of sugars.

STEVIA is my sweetener of choice. It is a perennial plant native to Paraguay and Brazil. The sweetness comes from the leaves which are crushed or distilled to create a powder or syrup. It can be purchased at health food stores, online and from larger supermarkets.

Stevia is a lot sweeter than traditional sugars so you only need to use a fraction. The ratios are as follows: 1 cup of sugar is the equivalent of about 1 teaspoon stevia liquid or powder, and 1 tablespoon of sugar is the equivalent of ¼ teaspoon powder or about 8 drops. A teaspoon of sugar equates to a pinch of powder or 2 drops of liquid.

SUGAR		STEVIA
1 cup	=	1 teaspoon liquid or powder
1 tablespoon	=	¼ teaspoon or about 8 drops
1 teaspoon	=	a pinch of powder or 2 drops of liquid

XYLITOL is a sugar substitute found naturally in fibrous fruits and veggies, such as plums and corn, and is also produced naturally in the body. Xylitol is metabolised slowly so it won't cause the 'sugar spikes' that can be experienced with other products. It can, however, cause stomach pain and also have a laxative effect when consumed in excess for some people with fructose malabsorption issues, so test it in small quantities first.

Xylitol also promotes oral health and reduces the incidence of tooth decay. And as an added benefit, a 2004 study found that xylitol damages Streptococcus pneumoniae, one of the main causes of ear infections, by destabilising the bacteria and thereby preventing it from multiplying.

It's a handy ingredient to use in baking and the ratio to sugar is 1 to 1. I recommend that you start by adding half that amount, doing a taste test, and adjusting accordingly.

RICE MALT SYRUP has the sweetness of caramelised honey. It is made by culturing rice with enzymes to break down the starches and then the mixture is cooked until it becomes a syrup. Due to its mixture of complex carbohydrates, maltose and a small amount of glucose, it provides a steady supply of energy to the body. Use the same quantity of rice malt syrup as you would sugar.

COCONUT SUGAR has low glycaemic index (GI) so does not cause sugar spikes. Although it does contain fructose, it has other health benefits that make it a suitable sugar substitute. It's derived from the sap of the coconut palm flower and contains minerals and amino acids such as glutamic acids, an important component in metabolism and which also acts as a neurotransmitter. Again, you can use it in the same quantity as you would regular sugar.

DEXTROSE is a simple monosaccharide found in plants and cells. You can purchase it as a powder and use it in baking. A word of caution: dextrose has a very high glycaemic index (GI). It raises blood sugar levels and stimulates a high insulin response very quickly. Divide the amount of sugar by 0.7 to get the quantity of dextrose required as a substitute.

AGAVE can also be used as a sugar substitute, although I don't recommend it as it is 90% fructose and highly processed. When fructose is metabolised by the body, the fatty acids accumulate as fat in your liver and muscle tissues, leading to insulin resistance, which can then progress to metabolic syndrome and Type II diabetes. The metabolism of fructose by your liver creates waste products and toxins, including a hefty amount of uric acid, which switches on your fat lever, resulting in weight gain.

AGING ACCELERATORS

There is a multitude of aging accelerators which can put you on a high-speed journey to looking and feeling 100 years older than you actually are. One of the major factors that control the speed at which you age is the functionality of your digestive system.

If you subject your body to crash diets, your gut will become sluggish and overworked, and your body unable to absorb the nutrients it needs to function. This results in different areas of your body – such as your skin and nails, hair, muscles and bones – becoming undernourished. You could be eating the healthiest foods on the planet but without a healthy digestive system, you will be unable to absorb their goodness and reap the benefits.

To improve bad digestion, it's essential to rule out any allergies. You could start with an elimination diet to work out what your body doesn't like, and then try a simple diet of foods which are easy to digest. You might want to have one day a week where you eat mineral-rich bone broths or nutrient-rich green soups to give your digestive system a rest.

Taking probiotics can be helpful if you have an imbalance of gut bacteria. Once your gut is sorted you'll be able to break down food so that you can benefit internally and externally from their nutrients, which will provide you with nourishment and energy.

Other ways to improve your digestion are to eat less and stop before you're completely full – it takes 20 minutes for your brain to know your stomach is full, which is important to remember when you are tempted to go back for a second helping. It's also a good idea to try not to eat less than two to three hours before going to bed, and eat and chew your food well, slowly and mindfully. Always listen to your body and the signals it sends you.

Unnecessary inflammation is another accelerator. As we age, our body's inflammatory response can become overactive, leading to activated immune cells. This puts stress on our immune systems. Many researchers believe that systemic inflammation is due, in part, to modern lifestyles: our diets, sedentary jobs and exposure to environmental pollutants like tobacco smoke and exhaust fumes.

Anti-inflammatory foods to include in your diet are those rich in omega-3, such as sardines, mackerel, salmon and tuna; and good fats, such as flaxseed oil and chia oil. See page 26 for more information on anti-inflammatory foods.

Oxidation also causes premature aging. It occurs when cells become highly reactive and combine with other molecules, resulting in oxidative stress and free radicals. Free radicals cause collagen breakdown, which leads to wrinkles. Some other culprits that cause oxidative stress include alcohol, UV light and chemicals in food and cleaning products. Antioxidant foods to include in your diet are kidney, pinto or adzuki beans or small red beans. Rich in flavonoids, these foods help reduce inflammation.

Hormone imbalance can also affect the aging process – when your hormones are out of alignment you can sleep badly, put on weight, develop allergies and cravings and your skin can start to wrinkle. Some of the effects of an imbalance of thyroid hormones are fatigue, dry skin, cold hands and feet, thinning hair, brittle nails, weight gain/fluid retention, menstrual irregularities and loss of libido. To redress the imbalance, eat more brown rice, quinoa, pepitas (pumpkin seeds), nuts and oysters. If you're concerned about your hormones, have a chat to your doctor about it.

Another aging accelerator is excess acidity in the body. Cells in the body function better when they are slightly alkaline. If you're eating too many acid-forming foods – such as grain-fed meats, coffee, cheese and fatty foods – you'll be more susceptible to the aging process. Green juices are the perfect antidote to an overly acidic system.

A good point to remember for a beautiful you is that a strict diet where you eliminate certain foods altogether is often not a good idea. Restricting your intake of specific foods, rather than eliminating them altogether, is going to yield more results. Cut back as much as possible on acid-forming, pro-inflammatory foods. Finding foods that are easy for you to digest is your essential goal. This may mean that you cannot eat too much raw food or an ingredient that may be troubling you.

TOP SEVEN FOODS FOR LONGEVITY

It's never too late to start consuming high-nutrient, antioxidant-rich, clean and unadulterated foods to contribute to your health. The effects of eating close to nature are cumulative and influence not only your health, but your emotional state and general wellbeing. Take some time to think about the food you are eating, not just in terms of preparation or taste but also how it was grown, where it came from and whether it's in season. Reform your personal food chain – not only will you look and feel better, the planet will thank you.

Indulge in SOLE food by choosing foods which are Sustainable, Organic, Local and Ethical.

Slow down the passage of time with these highly beneficial, nutritious foods. Here are my Top Seven Foods for Longevity.

BERRIES: High in protective plant antioxidants and containing phytochemicals and colour pigments called anthocyanins, berries get a big thumbs up as a beauty-booster. The phytochemicals found in berries have been associated with healthy aging and increase the potency of your intake of Vitamin C. Berries are very good sources of quercetin, a flavonol that has two important jobs in the body. Quercetin works as an anti-carcinogen and an antioxidant, which means it can protect the body and lower the risk of certain cancers. It also promotes urinary tract health. Berries have anti-inflammatory properties and researchers report that they also help slow down the loss of mental function that can be associated with aging. A word of caution: they can also be high in pesticides so try to go organic. Include cranberries, raspberries, strawberries and blueberries in your diet a few times a week.

WILD SALMON: A great source of omega-3 fats – the ultimate anti-aging nutrient – and healthy fat which can fend off heart disease, improve your skin and reverse sun damage. Wild salmon is an excellent source of Vitamin D and selenium for healthy hair, skin, nails and bones. Nutritionists advise eating two servings a week which can provide you with Vitamin B12 and regulate your blood pressure.

NUTS: Containing healthy oils, fibre, vitamins, minerals, potent phytochemicals and the amino acid arginine, nuts are also a good protein-rich snack. The best nuts for aging gracefully are almonds and brazil nuts. Nuts are a rich source of alpha-linolenic

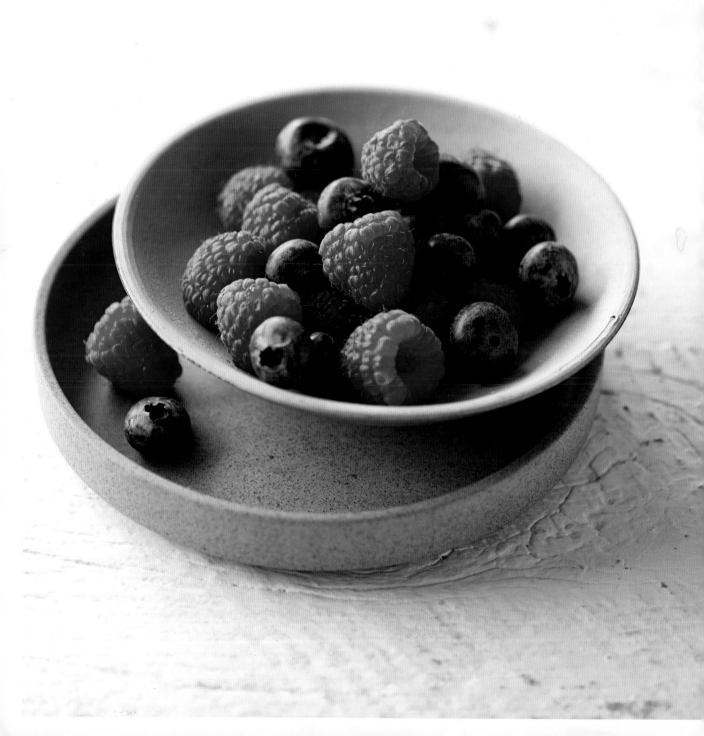

acid (ALA), the precursor to the omega-3 fatty acids DHA and EPA, which are great anti-inflammatories. Nuts are a great skin food too – you only need a small amount of almonds to improve your skin and make it glow as they contain Vitamin E. Eat a small handful (around 15–20) a day.

Swap out expensive skin treatments for berries, replace complexion creams with dark leafy greens, include wild salmon for reversing sun damage and use garlic to ease bloating and rub out wrinkles.

DARK LEAFY GREENS: Bursting with health benefits, spinach and leafy greens are a must-have food, and the darker, the better. They deliver a huge amount of Vitamin A which supports the turnover and production of new skin cells. They contain all sorts of goodies, including a selection of phytonutrients and antioxidants, Vitamins K, C and E, folate, and carotenoids as well as the top four essential minerals – calcium, magnesium, iron and potassium. Greens to include in your diet are spinach, cos (romaine) lettuce, kale and silverbeet (Swiss chard). Try to eat at least two cups a day. Juicing is a great way to boost your intake of greens.

SARDINES: These little guys are my favourite go-to meal and they are sky-high in omega-3 fatty acids. The good news is they contain almost no mercury and are loaded with minerals such as calcium, iron, magnesium, potassium and zinc. They're inexpensive and easy to bring to the table. They're good for the brain, hair, skin and nails.

Protein also contributes to maintaining youthful skin, and sardines supply quality protein. I eat a tin a day but if you're not a sardine lover then try tuna, salmon or mackerel. Not a fish fan? Swap out your oil for flaxseed, chia or extra virgin olive.

'When flaxseed becomes a normal part of the diet, a culture will achieve greater health.'
MAHATMA GANDHI (1869-1948)

FLAXSEEDS: A nifty little longevity secret and an abundant natural source of alpha-linolenic acid. This acid is one of the primary omega-3 fatty acids which is vital for decreasing inflammation. Flaxseeds contain insoluble dietary fibre, which helps in the promotion of more regular bowel movements and the removal of toxins from the body, promoting digestive health. Add a tablespoon of seeds to smoothies, sprinkle ground flaxseeds into cereal, soups and homemade baked goods, or scatter on top of vegetables. Flaxseed oil tastes delicious on salads too.

GARLIC: Such an amazing all-rounder and I've included it in many of the recipes. Not only does it have strong life-extension properties, it's also a powerful antibacterial, antifungal and antiviral agent, a potent blood thinner and it's full of antioxidants. Garlic promotes the growth of white blood cells, the body's natural germ fighters. Both fresh and dried garlic have been shown to lower harmful LDL cholesterol and high blood pressure. Garlic is a miracle food that can successfully diminish signs of aging due to its formidable properties as an antioxidant. The antioxidant components of garlic can protect the skin against damage caused by oxidation, and environmental stressors, and therefore prevents skin from becoming wrinkly. Eat daily with gusto!

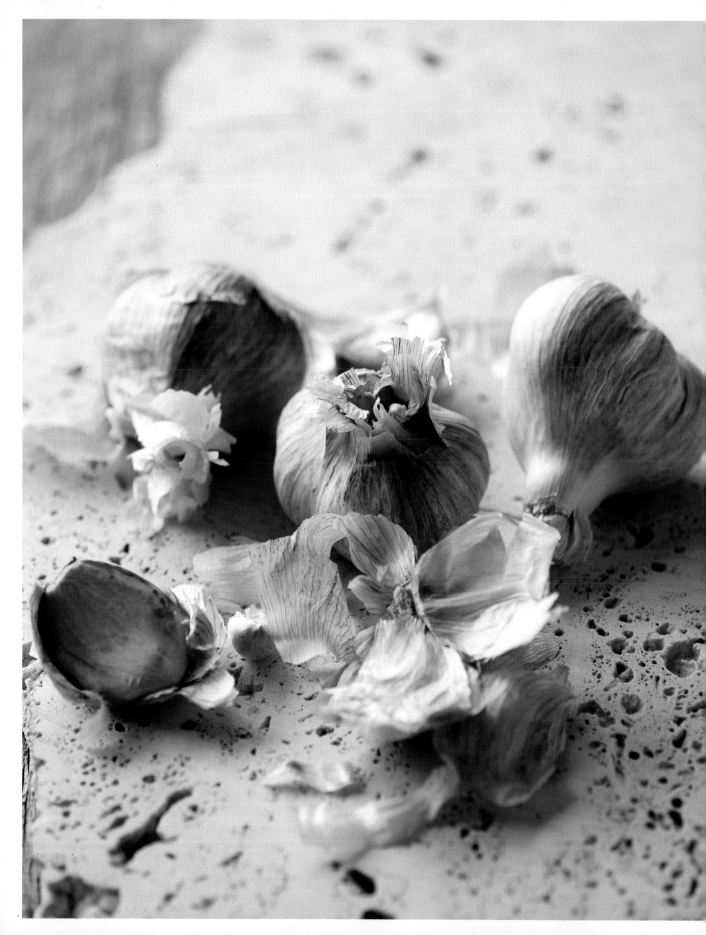

COMMON BEAUTY CONCERNS RECTIFIED WITH FOOD

Did you know?

Every 28 days your skin replaces itself.

Your surface lung cells renew every 21 days.

Your liver cells have a life span of 150 days.

Your bone-building cells can renew completely in 10 years.

And how does this happen?

Your body makes these new cells from the food that you eat.

What you eat becomes you.

So let's all make good choices about what we put into our bodies.

Following are some common beauty problems and the foods that you can eat to solve them.

BRITTLE HAIR AND DRY/FLAKY SCALP: No-one wants to look like Scarecrow from *The Wizard of Oz*. To keep your hair shiny and your scalp healthy, include a variety of vitamins and minerals in your diet. Eat foods high in folic acid, which is found in asparagus, broccoli, avocado, chickpeas and lentils, and foods that contain Vitamin B12, which is found in animal proteins such as chicken, oysters, egg and fish. Eating real butter and egg yolks will provide you with a supply of Vitamin A. Copper from shellfish, beans and nuts, and zinc in grass-fed meats and leafy green vegetables are perfect foods to include for strong, shiny hair and a flake-free scalp. Eat these regularly for glamorous shine and a dazzling glow and say goodbye to bad hair days forever.

RED EYES: Do you sometimes get home after a long day of staring at a computer screen with the AC on high only to feel like a vampire from *Twilight*? If this is the case, unless you're out partying or watching a Meg Ryan tear jerker, red eyes will clear up after the body has naturally had a chance to recuperate and rest. But here's a word of warning: enter the dark world of eye drop abusers and at some point down the road, you'll learn a lesson the tough way. Using eye drops and eye whiteners will temporarily relieve eye redness as they narrow blood vessels in your eyes. While this takes the redness out for about 2 hours, eventually rebound redness will rear its ugly head, and the more you use the drops, the redder your eyes will become. The best way to alleviate this is to stop using drops altogether. You may have continuing redness for a few weeks but over time your eyes will recover. Bloodshot eyes, however, can be the result of drinking alcohol or eating a nutritionally poor diet. Avoid bloodshot eyes by filling up on filtered water, wearing sunglasses when outside and eating plenty of fresh fruits and vegetables, especially those rich in flavonoids such as brightly coloured berries.

BLOATING: Everyone feels a little bloated from time to time but if you're bloated regularly, you may want to have a closer look at your diet and digestion. Bloating can also be a sign of a bigger health issue and be disruptive to your life. You might have trouble fitting into your normal clothes and have to unbutton your pants on a regular basis or it may just make you feel lethargic, sluggish and generally under the weather.

It might sound contradictory but boosting your water intake and using probiotics will help to bring the gut back into balance and diminish the bloating. Water helps keep your digestion moving so air doesn't become trapped inside. Foods that are high in fibre are equally important. I recommend that you eat smaller meals, quit drinking soft drinks and using artificial sweeteners, reduce your intake of fried foods and sodium, and start the day off with a healthy nut and seed muesli made with almond milk and topped with flaxseed and chia seeds. You might want to try my delicious Cranberry and Walnut Granola on page 69. Herbal teas are also anti-bloating – try fennel, peppermint, ginger or chamomile.

SUN-DAMAGED SKIN: If your skin appears older than you, the top vitamins to boost it are Vitamins A, B2, B3, B6, B12, C and E. Delicious blackberries have all six and so adding them to your smoothie, cereal or salad is definitely beneficial. To boost your intake of Vitamin E, eat a handful of nuts – this in turn helps fight free radicals, which are generated by UV sunlight and damaged skin. Simply adding a handful of nuts like walnuts and almonds to your daily diet will boost your Vitamin E intake and help your skin retain moisture. Regular sunshine and the Vitamin D3 it produces is actually beneficial for the skin and hugely important for overall health, so the best tactic is to enjoy 20 minutes of sun a day for restoring Vitamin D levels and then cover up your face and delicate areas. Also topically try a squeeze of lemon juice or aloe vera on sun spots – it will lighten them naturally and over time you will be splotch-free.

WRINKLES/THIN SKIN: Wrinkles occur due to sun damage, dry skin, unhealthy lifestyle and aging. Keeping your skin moist and supple will keep you from looking like a fossil. Fish such as salmon has high protein content, a building block for great skin, and their omega-3 content will help your skin stay moist and youthful. Your skin will also benefit from the consumption of flaxseed. Opt for flaxseed oil or add ground flaxseed to your cereals or to smoothies. Sunflower seeds are rich in Vitamin E and selenium and will nourish your skin from the inside out and slow down the development of saggy, wrinkled skin. Sprinkle them on salads and eat as a snack. Don't reach for toxic night creams or wrinkle fighters from your bathroom cabinet, but rather apply coconut or avocado oil on your body and face and gently massage it in every night, 30 minutes before bedtime to let it soak in and awake with a natural glow.

PIGMENTATION: Blotchy and pigmented skin has a bad habit of catching the light in the most inappropriate and awkward places making you appear splodgy and older than your years. There are two types of pigmentation – hypopigmentation and hyperpigmentation – and these cover everything from sun spots, dark freckles and liver spots to larger areas of discolouration. Hypopigmentation is a decrease in skin tone, which is when patches of skin become lighter in colour than the normal surrounding skin. Hyperpigmentation is the opposite and quite common. Skin can become darker in colour than the normal surrounding skin and occurs when an excess of melanin, the brown pigment that produces normal skin colour, forms deposits in the skin. Pigmentation can occur due to a number of factors including genetics, sun exposure, stress, fluctuating hormones, menopause, insulin resistance and excessive exposure to chemicals in skincare products and hair dyes. If you scour the ingredients lists of everyday skin creams you'll notice that many of them contain Vitamin A. Our bodies convert beta-carotene into this skin-brightening vitamin, which helps prevent cell damage and premature aging. For a gentler and more wallet-friendly pigmentation prevention method which will see you go from patchy to perfect in a flash, load up on orange and green veggies, such as pumpkin, sweet potato, carrots, spinach, kale, and broccoli.

DARK CIRCLES AND PUFFY EYES: Unless you're Alice Cooper, dark puffy eyes are hard to pull off and even harder to conceal. This is a very common condition and about two-thirds of the female population suffer from it. Dark circles which creep in under the eyes are caused by tiny blood vessels showing through the delicate skin that surrounds the eye. As we age, the skin becomes thinner and more translucent, making the problem more evident. Dark circles can appear even worse when there are additional eye bags or puffiness, which is caused by an accumulation of fluid in the delicate tissues surrounding the eye. Using heavy toxic overnight eye creams and eye-care products just thin the skin and paradoxically make them puff up even more because the oils in the creams cause fluid to stay in the eye area. Eating too much salt can contribute to water retention and create dark, puffy

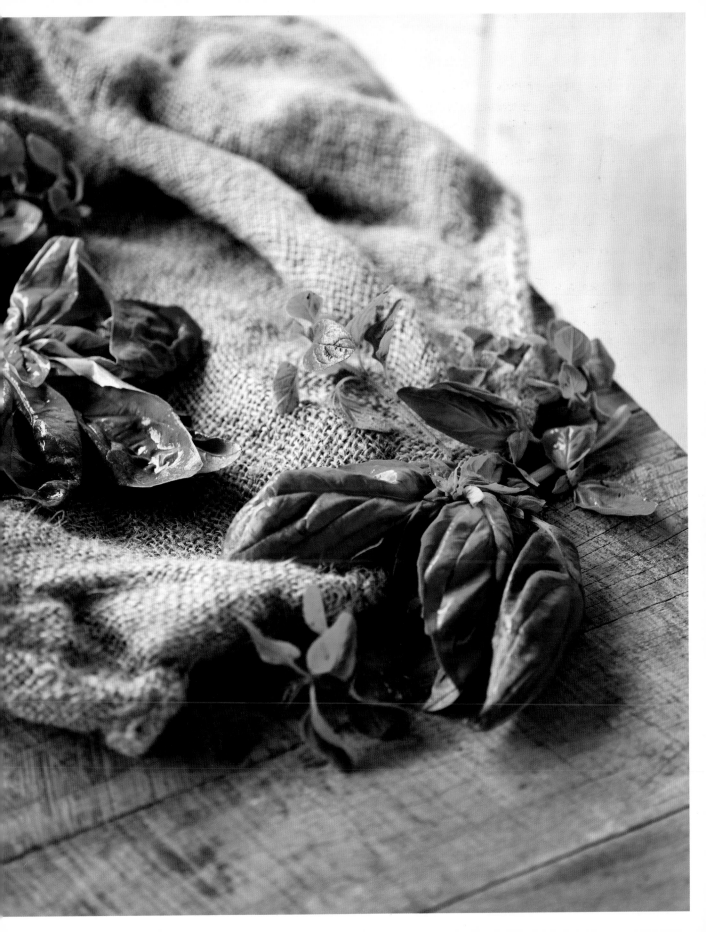

eyes. To counteract this, load up on natural diuretics to help flush your system. Foods such as cucumber and celery can help. And, drink, drink, drink, drink filtered water.

LOOSE SKIN: If your sagging jaw line has more floppy jowls than a St Bernard, then you might want to try boosting your Vitamins C and A intake. Vitamin C aids in the body's production of collagen, which is a basic part of the structure of your skin. As you age, your skin starts to lose firmness as its fatty tissue disappears and its production of strengthening collagen and elastin slows down. It's best to avoid too much fruit that is high in fructose, so opt for other foods rich in Vitamin C such as red and green chillies, capsicum (peppers), dark leafy greens like kale, fresh parsley and broccoli. Foods rich in Vitamin A include carrots, sweet potatoes and egg yolks.

ACNE: Although genetics and other factors may play a part in the appearance of your skin, being aware of what you eat can improve skin quality, and reduce blemishes. Acne can affect all ages. It's more prolific in teens to thirty-somethings but adult acne is now on the rise. If you reach for an acne treatment you'll more often than not find that the little handy hints booklet is accompanied by the words, 'If irritation occurs consult your doctor', which will then result in you being handed a prescription for antibiotics or hormonal treatments such as the contraceptive pill. If you prefer to go down the natural road, foods that contain zinc, such as seafood and flaxseed oil, can help fight acne because zinc is involved in the metabolising of testosterone, which affects the production of sebum, an oil that is released from the skin and is a primary cause of acne.

DETOXING YOUR SKIN

You don't need to go on a five-day fast, use hardcore expulsion methods or rearrange your internal furniture in order to simply detoxify your skin. The skin is often referred to as 'the third kidney', due to its role in removing waste from the body. The condition and quality of your skin is therefore a mirror for what's really happening inside.

Ultimately, if you want to achieve gorgeous, glowing skin, you'll need to decrease your toxic load by choosing organic, chemical-free vegetables; avoiding additives and preservatives in foods; drinking high-quality filtered water; and eliminating chemically-laden beauty and household cleaning products from your home. These are just a few simple steps that you can incorporate into your life that will significantly reduce the toxic burdens on your body; and as a result, your skin will be free to shine, rather than being overburdened by detoxification duties.

Unless you live in a bubble, it's virtually impossible to avoid *all* toxins that life presents to us. They're pretty much everywhere around us, even in the air we breathe. It's boring to get really hung up on avoiding every toxin around us but there are some simple, easy and cost-effective ways to detox. By adopting these 'detoxification rituals' as part of your everyday lifestyle, you'll notice that your skin is also detoxified. Your eyes will become whiter and brighter, and your complexion will radiate on a whole new level.

One of the first things that I do when I wake up in the morning, after my hot water and lemon, is dry body brushing. It's an invigorating way to jump-start the day and provides some serious detoxification. It does so by activating the lymph system, your body's transit scheme for food and oxygen to be transported through the blood into your cells, and then for your cells to return waste back into your bloodstream. By dry body brushing daily, you are increasing and improving the movement of the lymph system so that waste is eliminated and nutrients are delivered to the skin cells at a higher capacity. This will strengthen, exfoliate and improve moisture levels in the skin, as well as alleviate vein and lymph congestion; or what's commonly known as cellulite. Buying a quality brush with dry plant bristles will bring optimum results. Start at your feet, and always do the left hand side of your body first to get your circulation going. Use long, quick, sweeping strokes of the brush upwards, and in towards the heart.

Since following a more anti-inflammatory diet for my fibromyalgia, I have also found that incorporating gentle exercise into my routine has helped to control my muscle aches and stiffness and also benefited my body in a detoxification sense. Exercise creates the conditions under which the body is forced to breathe deeply, increase circulation and excrete sweat. It improves detoxification simply by getting the detoxifying organs and systems 'moving'. The lymph system, unlike the circulatory system, doesn't have an inbuilt 'pump', and therefore relies on body brushing, massage and bodily movement to get it functioning. Digestive function is also improved through exercise; it will function more optimally and regularly with consistent physical movement. Walking, light jogging, swimming, bike riding, yoga and pilates are all ideal exercise options. Housework is a great example of incidental exercise. Everyday exercise is what counts the most.

Detox naturally by getting your antioxidants from foods such as berries, red capsicum (peppers), beans and artichokes.

By eating particular foods, we can find other ways to detoxify and cleanse our skin from the inside out. Eating gelatinous plant foods including chia seeds, seaweeds and even aloe vera is especially beneficial, as these all contain gel-like substances that move through our digestive tract, absorbing toxins and depositing them into the colon. The benefit of this process is that these toxins are dealt with in the digestive system, and therefore have no chance of working their way into our skin cells. Chia seeds can be easily incorporated into your diet, and as they don't have an overpowering and specific taste they blend into most dishes quite well. Add them to smoothies, omelettes, your morning porridge or muesli, or simply soak a tablespoon in your morning glass of water for a few minutes and drink it down.

❱SUPERCHARGED TIP❰

A green juice a day keeps the dermatologist away.

Organic green vegetables are highly detoxifying, but it can be incredibly difficult to chow down on enough spinach and celery to get a highly effective result. That's where your juicer will come in handy, particularly in the mornings when you want to have something nutritious on the run. In just one glass of juice, you can consume a huge amount of green vegetables, and with the fibrous content removed, the powerful cocktail of vitamins, minerals, antioxidants, phytonutrients and enzymes will be able to penetrate your bloodstream within minutes. Green juices cleanse, purify and oxygenate the blood; increasing circulation and flushing harmful toxins from your organs. Adding herbs such as parsley and coriander (cilantro) will really supercharge your juice's detoxification capabilities. Coriander binds with heavy metals, releasing them from the body and parsley contains potent amounts of chlorophyll, which acts as an excellent cleanser for your entire system, including the skin.

When it comes to rituals, you don't need to give up your daily cuppa Joe altogether, but replacing your daily grind with dandelion root tea will really help. Dandelion tea has incredible liver detox capabilities while coffee is dehydrating, acid forming, nutrient depleting, adrenal stressing and burdens the liver, our major detoxifying organ. Cleansing your body with dandelion tea will allow the liver to do its primary job, which is breaking down toxins and allowing them to be excreted through the colon and through your urine. This will leave you feeling more energised, motivated and looking beautiful, because your toxins are being filtered out efficiently.

ANTI-INFLAMMATORY FOODS

Most of us are familiar with inflammation on the surface of our bodies, which involves local redness, heat, swelling and pain, but there is another kind of inflammation that lingers within our bodies. Inflammation exists within us all and is an extremely powerful, necessary function for our survival. It's the cornerstone of the body's healing response; ensuring that appropriate nourishment and adequate immune activity are delivered to an area that is injured or under attack.

However, there's a darker side to the wonderful healing capabilities of inflammation and because of its gripping, powerful responsiveness, inflammation can be incredibly destructive to your health, particularly when it extends beyond the boundaries of a localised area, or continues for long periods of time.

The body has very complex mechanisms to ensure that inflammation stays where it's supposed to stay, and ends where it's supposed to end, but it's becoming increasingly common that people have persistent inflammation lingering in their bodies. Unlike a normal, healthy inflammatory response, this type of inflammation serves no purpose.

Foods that contribute to inflammation in the body are saturated fats from poorly fed animals and animals fed and finished on genetically modified corn and grains, antibiotics and hormones. Trans-fats from margarine, shortening and hydrogenated oils are also huge contributors. When it comes to eating fats and oils, it's important to avoid a diet high in omega-6 and low in omega-3 fatty acids, as this unhealthy balance leads to an increase in cytokines, proteins released in the cells that trigger inflammation.

Sugar is a major factor in inflammation, as well as any form of refined food. Refined grains that can be found in your everyday, supermarket breakfast cereals, breads, pasta and muesli bars are pro-inflammatory as the refining process depletes fibre and Vitamin B, which are needed to keep inflammation at bay.

Cruciferous vegetables have potent anti-inflammatory and anti-cancer effects, and include a range of vegetables such as broccoli, kale and cabbage. Bok choy (pak choy) boasts a particularly high anti-inflammatory effect due to its potent concentration of beta-carotene and Vitamin A. Interestingly, one serve of bok choy contains up to 70 mg of omega-3 fats. Omega-3s are paramount in reducing the body's inflammatory status, as well as preventing the risks and symptoms of a number of disorders influenced by inflammation. Other omega-3 rich foods include flaxseeds, walnuts, navy (haricot) beans, kidney beans and cold-water oily fish including salmon, mackerel, black cod, herring, anchovies and, my favourite, sardines.

The trusty sardine in particular offers a serious omega-3, inflammation-busting hit. These little swimmers are one of the most concentrated sources of the omega-3 fatty acids EPA and DHA as well as Vitamin B12, all of which have been found to decrease cardiovascular disease, one of the top inflammatory-related illnesses. The omega-3 fatty acids found in sardines lower triglycerides and unhealthy cholesterol levels, while Vitamin B12 keeps levels of homocysteine

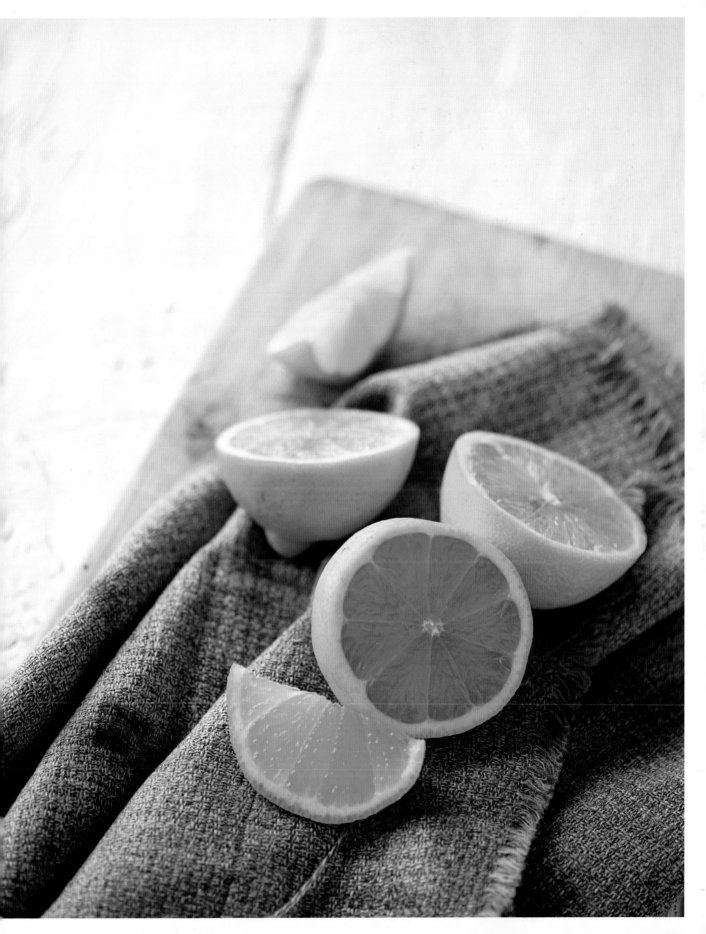

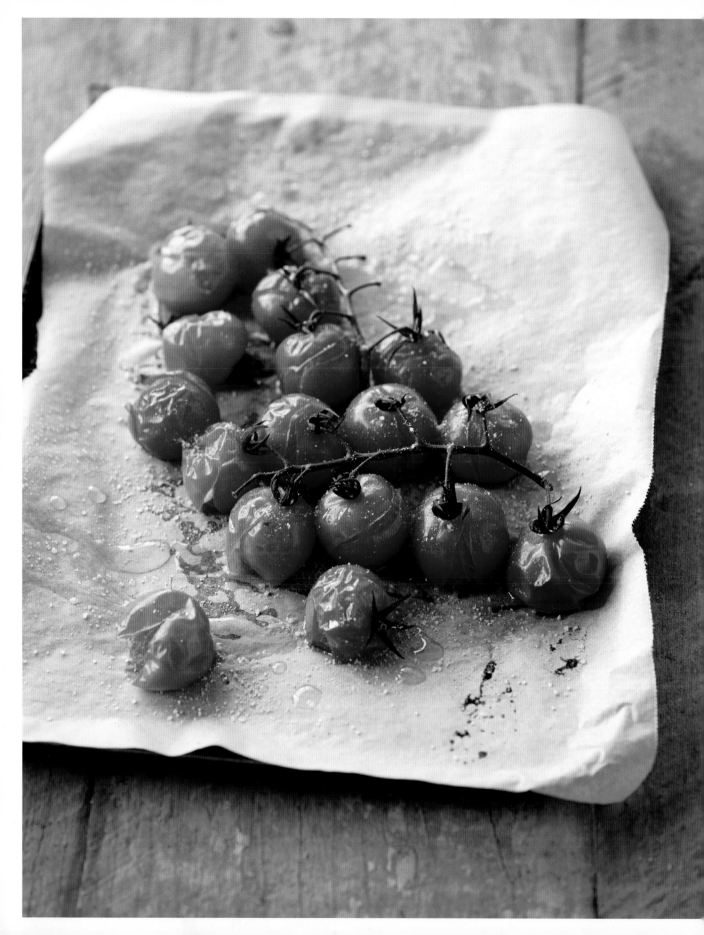

in balance. Homocysteine can damage artery walls, with elevated levels being directly linked to atherosclerosis. Tinned sardines in extra virgin olive oil are the most convenient option, as they require minimum preparation. You can add them to salads, or combine them with lemon juice, avocado, Celtic sea salt and cracked pepper on a gluten-free cracker for a tasty, nutrient-dense snack. Or you could also try the Seanuts recipe on page 99 for another delicious way to include sardines in your diet.

Adding a variety of herbs and spices to your pantry will not only pump up the flavour of your favourite meals, but will provide powerful anti-inflammatory benefits. Turmeric in particular has been recognised by scientists to hold incredible anti-inflammatory effects due to its active ingredient, curcumin. Turmeric has the ability to protect fats against oxidisation during the cooking process, as well as shielding the body against oxidative stress once the cooked meal has been consumed. Turmeric can be bought fresh, or dried in the form of a powder, and is a perfect ingredient to add to soups, curries and Indian-style dishes.

Ginger is the root of a plant from the same family as turmeric and has been used as a remedy for centuries in Asian, Indian and Arabic systems of medicine. This spicy ingredient is a potent anti-inflammatory, inhibiting the formation of inflammatory prostaglandins, thereby reducing the pain associated with osteoarthritis and other inflammatory illnesses. Studies reveal that ginger may help halt the inflammation that's associated with liver cancer by stopping the pro-inflammatory TNF-α protein. Include freshly grated ginger in stir-fries, soups and curries, or add it to hot water with lemon and a couple of drops of stevia to make a spicy, soothing tea. I like to drink this first thing in the morning before I eat anything as it is a wonderful internal alkaliserz and detoxer.

Another nutrient to really grab hold of for an anti-inflammatory diet is polyphenols. Extra virgin olive oil contains significant quantities of polyphenols. Researchers worldwide find that a diet rich in olive oil polyphenols is associated with healthier breast tissue, colon function, cardiovascular function, and provides protection from the inflammatory effects of secondary smoke and other environmental toxins. Remember to use cold-pressed extra virgin olive oil on salads and only heat it to a moderate temperature.

GOOD FATS FOR SUCCESSFUL AGING

'There is a fountain of youth: it is your mind, your talents, the creativity you bring to your life and the lives of people you love. When you learn to tap this source, you will truly have defeated age.'

SOPHIA LOREN

With daily wear and tear and damage to the skin and organs, visible aging is inevitable. Factors that contribute to how we visibly age include oxidative stress, glycation, telomere shortening, chronological age, genetics and lifestyle.

In our society, fat has been the target of much scorn, but it is absolutely necessary for graceful aging and a healthy youthful complexion. Consuming the right fats and oils supplies the essential fatty acids (EFAs) that our bodies are incapable of producing on their own, and these are highly important for preventing aging in the skin. The right kinds of fats will also ferry fat-soluble vitamins such as A, D, E and K around the body; delivering these much-needed nutrients to your skin cells, resulting in a healthy complexion. For a youthful appearance, it is best to include the following fats and oils in your diet regularly.

Omega-3 fats help reduce inflammation in the body, which researchers have touted to be a driving force behind chronic disease. Their studies reveal that omega-3s promote healthy levels of cholesterol and triglycerides, support normal blood pressure and help maintain healthy circulation and blood vessels. Sources of omega-3 fats include fish oil from salmon, tuna, halibut, mackerel, sardines, herring and other cold-water species. Omega-3s are responsible for skin repair, moisture content and skin elasticity. Krill oil is also beneficial – since I've been taking 1000 mg krill oil daily I have noticed an enormous reduction in my fibromyalgia symptoms.

Omega-3s can also be derived from our body's conversion of plant fats from sources such as flaxseed, walnuts, algae and pepita (pumpkin seeds). Flaxseed oil is one of the richest plant sources of alpha-linolenic acid (ALA), being comprised of over 50% of this essential omega-3 dietary fat. Interestingly, a wave of new studies point to the soothing and healing properties of flaxseed oil on the repair of inflamed intestines. This calming and anti-inflammatory effect helps to ensure the health of the gut, which is often mirrored in the health of the complexion. Eating flaxseed oil also helps to normalise the skin lipids and seal in moisture, resulting in plumper, more hydrated skin.

Making sure that you have the correct ratio of omega-3 to omega-6 fats is a strong factor in your successful aging blueprint. For many people this typically means an increase in your intake of omega-3 fats, and a decrease in your intake of omega-6 fats such as safflower, sunflower, corn, grapeseed and cottonseed oils. If you're wondering about which nuts to consume to balance out your ratio of fats, a handful of nuts every few days isn't going to make that much of a difference. Nuts with the lowest amount of omega-6s are macadamias, cashews, almonds, hazelnuts and pistachios. Nuts as a whole are found to reduce markers of systemic inflammation so don't get too hung up on the omega content of them if you're eating them in moderation.

OMEGA-6 CONTENT PER ¼ CUP NUTS	
Pine nuts	11.6 g
Walnuts	9.5 g
Brazil nuts	7.2 g
Pecans	5.8 g
Almonds	4.4 g
Pistachios	4.1 g
Hazelnuts	2.7 g
Cashews	2.6 g
Macadamias	0.5 g

WHICH OILS SHOULD I COOK WITH?

It's a good idea to familiarise yourself with the best oils to cook with and the ones which are better consumed unheated in their natural state. When an oil reaches its smoke point it changes its structure and becomes rancid. This means that in the process of fats and oils breaking down free radicals can be released, causing stress and damage on a cellular level throughout the body.

Coconut oil is one of the most beautifying oils that can be consumed. Although it's been feared in the past due to its high concentration of saturated fats, the unique medium chain structure of these fats, as well as the fact that they are plant-based and in a raw state, means that extra virgin coconut oil contains significant antiviral, antifungal and antimicrobial actions. Coconut oil is easily metabolised by the liver, and has antioxidant and anti-inflammatory properties that prevent aging in the skin. The lauric acid found in coconut oil is converted to monolaurin in the body, which fight the microbes that cause a range of skin infections. Organic extra virgin coconut oil is an exceptional internal beautifying oil, but can also be used as an

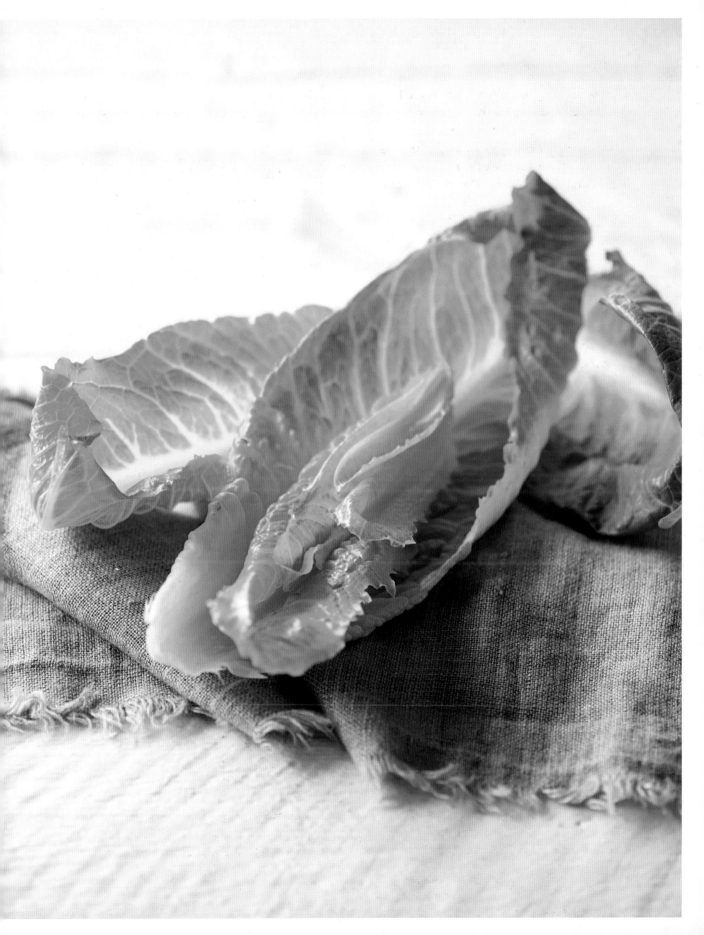

all-over face and body moisturiser, eye cream and hair oil.

Olive oil has long been recognised for its amazing health and beauty benefits. It contains high levels of monounsaturated fatty acids and antioxidants that have an anti-inflammatory effect on the body. It's an excellent source of Vitamin E, one of the most powerful antioxidants that helps to neutralise free radicals and prevent premature aging. Recent studies suggest that olive oil may be uniquely beneficial to skin due to the presence of polyphenol antioxidants and squalene. The best olive oil to consume is cold-pressed extra virgin.

Avocados are internal skin moisturisers. They're abundant in vitamins and minerals that are crucial to the health of your entire body. Particularly high in beta-carotene, lutein, Vitamins B6, C, E and K, selenium, zinc, folate, potassium and glutathione, avos are rich in healthy monounsaturated fats and omega-3 fatty acids, offering remarkable benefits to the human skin. They're high in carotenoid antioxidants, and contain the perfect amount and balance of dietary fats required for these antioxidants to be optimally absorbed. Included in this perfect balance is the presence of oleic acid, a monounsaturated fatty acid that helps the digestive tract to transport molecules that can carry carotenoids around the body. When combining an avocado with your salad, you are also maximising the uptake of these fat-soluble antioxidants into your skin cells, which are proven to fight against the free radicals that can cause aging. Studies show that eating avocados can help to increase the production of collagen, and reduce the size and appearance of wrinkles. It might sound outrageous but avocados can be dangerously addictive consumed first thing in the morning – I just pop half an avo into my morning juice for a creamy, thicker smoothie-like consistency. It will send your energy levels into overdrive, and fill you up too.

OILS WHICH CAN BE USED ON A HIGH HEAT:
Coconut oil
Avocado oil
Ghee
Organic butter
Sesame oil
Rice bran oil

MEDIUM TO LOW HEAT:
Extra virgin olive oil

BEST OILS TO BE CONSUMED COLD:
Extra virgin olive oil
Flaxseed oil
Macadamia oil
Hemp seed oil

TOP 20 BEAUTY-BOOSTING FOODS

Want to pump the brakes on unhealthy aging and look and feel your best? As you age, your body becomes less able to digest and absorb nutrients. This results in less nutrients actually making their way into your bloodstream and through to your skin. Choosing nutrient-rich foods which have a far greater concentration of body- and skin-beautifying nutrients will provide you with a free pass to receive more goodness and benefit from the results. With a few small nutritional tweaks to your diet, you can use everyday foods instead of topical solutions.

Why not ditch the skin perfectors and toners in favour of these foods and allow them to be an intrinsic part of your everyday skin routine.

Salmon is a wonder food full of omega-3s. It boosts the glow, suppleness, thickness and radiance of your skin.

Almonds contain Vitamin E and can help protect your skin from damaging UV rays. They're also an easy nibble when you're running around.

Flaxseeds can help prevent dry skin and reduce

the severity of psoriasis or eczema. High in fibre and omega-3s, flaxseed will keep your skin plumped and smooth.

Anchovies are high in omega-3s and these little fish add flavour and goodness to almost everything.

Mangoes and papayas have loads of Vitamins C and E, flavonoids and beta-carotene. Mangoes can help maintain a clear complexion, free of pimple breakouts.

Sweet potatoes will add lustre to your locks. Your body converts the beta-carotene in this food to Vitamin A, which is necessary for cell growth and renewal, and can keep your hair strong and shiny.

Kale is loaded with lutein, which keeps your eyes sparkling (and healthy) as well as Vitamin C, which is vital for skin health.

Coconut oil is the perfect oil to use topically as well as to add to your cooking to keep your skin soft and moist and maintain a youthful glow.

Tuna has crazy-high levels of selenium, a nutrient that helps prevent cellular damage.

Carrots are rich in Vitamin A, which is essential for smooth, shiny hair and supple skin.

Tomatoes contain lycopene, which helps protect skin against damage from the sun.

Cacao powder is loaded with antioxidants, magnesium and iron. This powder helps your skin's circulation and will help prevent a dull, sagging appearance.

Mussels are a great source of protein, Vitamins B and C, folate and zinc – all of which are needed for healthy skin and hair.

Blueberries are abundant in powerful antioxidants that help fight the free radicals in your body that may otherwise damage your skin.

Chia is another brilliant source of omega-3s. It is a superfood that works for you both inside and out.

Oysters don't just crank up your sex drive, the zinc prevalent in oysters can help fight breakouts and clear up dry skin.

Grass-fed beef is iron rich and can help prevent dark circles forming under your eyes and keep your skin from looking pale. It's also wonderful for improving hair quality and lustre.

Eggs are another source of iron that will help your skin glow and prevent dark circles around the eyes.

Water is essential to keep your skin hydrated.

SWAP OUTS

Now for the fun part – look at your current diet and do a few swap outs to make it a dynamic, successful-aging eating plan, which is going to make a big difference to the way you feel inside.

Food swaps don't need to be ominous. There are healthier versions of everyday foods which are wiser choices and ones which will make you feel your best. Eating yourself beautiful is not about restricting your food intake or going on a fad diet, if you have the thought that a food is banned you'll only end up craving that very food. Try these swaps for size:

- Never buy iceberg lettuce again! Fill your sandwich or salad bowl with baby spinach or finely chopped kale instead.
- Swap white potatoes for cauliflower, turnip or sweet potatoes when roasting or mashing.
- Add a spoonful of cacao powder to your morning breakfast shake.
- Sprinkle flaxseeds on top of your cereal or salads.
- Add smoked salmon to the top of your salad.
- Use flaxseed, chia or extra virgin olive oil instead of canola oil.
- Cut back on coffee by substituting it with dandelion tea.
- Use coconut oil and coconut flour when baking and give packaged flour the flick.
- Make breakfast the most powerful meal of your day: instead of packaged cereal, add a handful of walnuts, almonds and brazil nuts, flaxseeds, chia seeds, a scoop of sheep's milk yoghurt and almond milk to rolled oats and top it off with a handful of berries.

- Remember eggs aren't just for breakfast. Why not slice boiled egg on top of a spinach and kale salad, and top it with sardines and anchovies.
- Swap your soft drink for water. Always.
- When making lasagne, substitute pasta for thinly sliced zucchini (courgettes).
- Say no to unhealthy spreads and margarines and instead use real butter, avocado or nut butters.
- Keep grated carrot in an airtight container in your fridge. Add a handful to everything – your sandwich, your dinner plate, your snack plate.
- Swap the unhealthy biscuit for some healthy nuts when you need a 3 pm pick-me-up.
- Ditch the fat-laden and sugar-filled crackers and use flax crackers instead when you're enjoying a quick dip.
- Find places to squeeze in lentils – they pair well with salads or added to a meat sauce.
- Make seafood burgers with a fish high in omega-3s such as salmon or swordfish. Toss in some anchovies or sardines to boost the goodness.
- Swap hot chocolate made with whole milk for a hot chocolate made with cacao powder and almond milk.
- End each meal with something that crunches – some crisp berries, or carrot or celery sticks.

SUPER SKIN, HAIR AND NAILS

'Nature gives you the face you have at twenty; it is up to you to merit the face you have at fifty.'

COCO CHANEL (1883–1971)

The first barometer of your body's health is your skin and it can demonstrate how well you really are inside. Eating foods that nourish your body and eliminating those that are toxic or contribute no real nutrition will bring about a radical change in the appearance of your skin and overall health. When you think of an image of a beautiful person, chances are you're envisaging someone with shiny, bouncy, goddess-like hair; clear, glowing, radiant skin; and well-manicured, strong nails. This is no surprise, as beautiful looking skin, hair and nails are all an indication of vibrant health. Because we've been indoctrinated for so long by advertising and marketing, the way we aim to achieve gorgeousness in these three areas is through the empty promises of conventional beauty products. There is a growing awareness, however, that creating beauty from the inside out through a diet of real, whole foods is a more viable option. There is a growing movement of people who are becoming wise to the ingredients of toxic beauty products and the effects that they have on our bodies.

Have you noticed those white Thai young coconuts popping up in cafés, health food stores and even supermarkets? They may be the fruit du jour with hipsters but for very good reason. Not only are they a delicious, tropical delicacy, they're also bursting with complexion-boosting properties. The water within young coconuts is isotonic, meaning that it contains the same electrolyte concentration as the human body. It contains five essential electrolytes

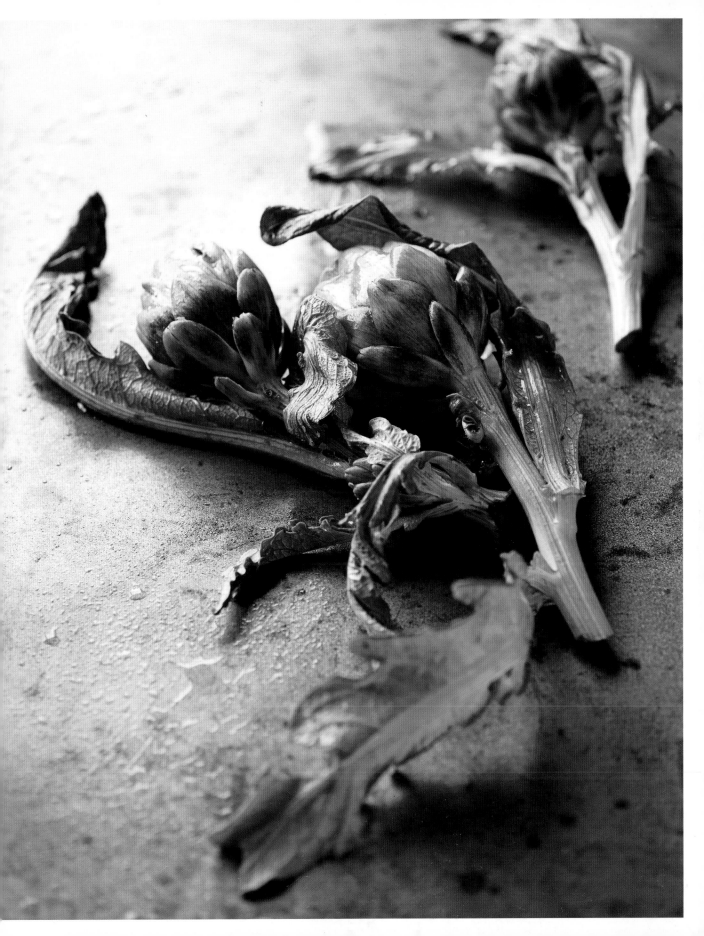

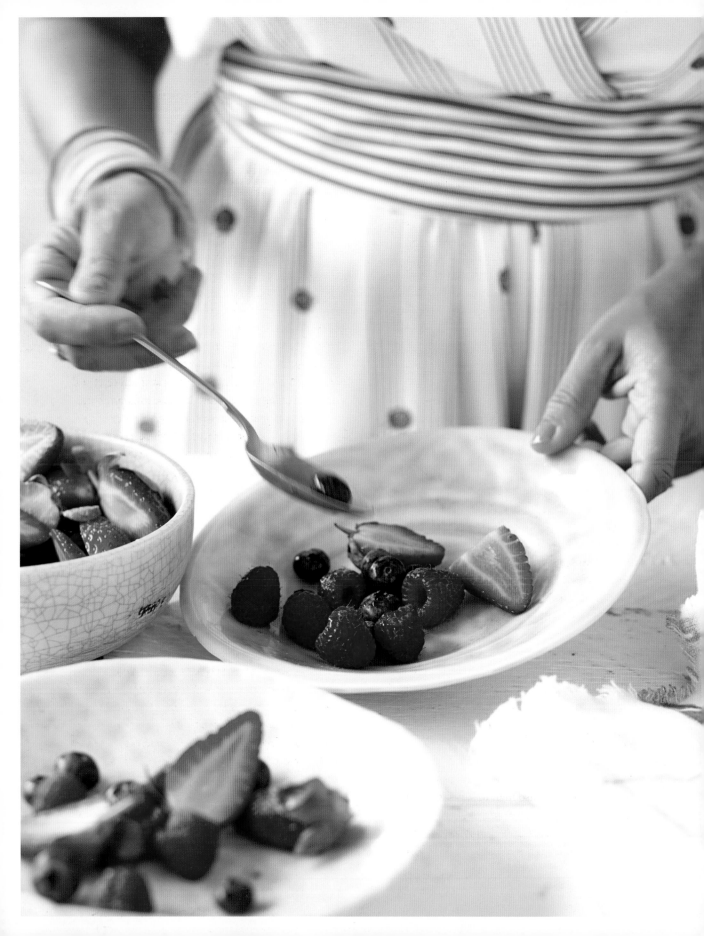

– potassium, magnesium, sodium, calcium and phosphorus. Consuming coconut water on a regular basis results in toxin elimination, replenishment of the system with vital minerals, and it significantly rehydrates the body, revealing a plumper, more hydrated complexion.

The flesh of the young coconut is bursting with medium chain beauty fats to nourish, protect and moisturise the skin from within, so using both the water and the flesh in smoothies, curries and desserts is a jazzy way to keep your skin in tip-top shape. For a concentrated dose of these fats, another wonderful complexion-boosting product is the organic, cold-pressed, extra virgin oil of the coconut. As previously discussed, this is a highly beautifying oil to consume as part of your diet, as well as applying externally.

Eating, blending and juicing your greens is a top-notch way to fill your body with the enzymes, vitamins, minerals and phytonutrients required for glowing, flawesome skin. Vegetables like my favourite kale, English spinach, celery and lettuce receive their vibrant green colour from chlorophyll; a nutrient-rich pigment that is highly detoxifying. Chlorophyll cleanses the body of harmful toxins that would otherwise cause hormone imbalances and skin problems. It also oxygenates the blood, alkalises the body and improves circulation to increase nutrient supply to the skin cells. Greens are also full of fibre, which help to keep the gut healthy, and the bowels busy at work removing toxins in the digestive tract. Healthy digestion and regular bowel movements are very important for the health of your complexion, and greens are a textbook way to keep this detoxification pathway flowing. Ongoing cleansing is vital to reaching your highest potential of health and beauty, and consuming loads of green, organic vegetables will guarantee this transpires.

While fruits may be full of vitamins and antioxidants, they're also high in sugar, which can lead to insulin spikes, hormonal upsets and an overproduction of sebum. This has been linked to being a cause and aggravator of acne and blemishes and dreaded snake skin. Thankfully, berries are a delicious, lower-sugar fruit option that boast a range of complexion-enhancing properties. They are high in Vitamin C, an important nutrient that helps the skin's collagen production. They're also brimming with a variety of antioxidants that protect against free radical damage that causes wrinkles. Eating a variety of different coloured berries will expose your cells to the multitude of different antioxidants that they all have to offer, and investing in some of the 'superfood' berries like goji, maqui or acai in the form of organic, raw powders is a way to really supercharge your skin health. Add these superfood berry powders, or different varieties of fresh organic berries, to your juices, smoothies, breakfasts or simply as a snack to detoxify the kidneys, cleanse the blood and pack a giant antioxidant punch that'll delay the aging process and decrease inflammation.

Our skin, just like any other organ in our body, is made up of cells with a high percentage of water. Adequate water intake is crucial for healthy digestion, circulation, enhancing nutrient uptake and ensuring healthy detoxification. Therefore it makes sense that the amount and quality of water you drink each day have an impact on the function and appearance of your skin. Commit to drinking at least a litre (35 fl oz/4 cups) of water a day, and more if you drink caffeinated beverages. I drink filtered water as I prefer not to have chlorine and chlorination by-products lurking in my system. Invest in a good-quality water filter jug, or one that is attached to your tap, and be sure to avoid drinking water out of plastic bottles, as they contain chemicals such as BPA that mimic and negatively affect hormone balance, which will in turn contribute to skin problems. By increasing the quality and having an adequate quantity of water each day you will increase the hydration of your skin, making it more resilient, and less prone to dryness, flakiness and wrinkles.

Rather than seeking a silicone-coating, chemical-rich cocktail in a bottle to answer the cry of lifeless hair, why not begin to fill your body with the most amazing, delicious wholefoods that will deliver a genuine, lasting result?

Vitamin E is one of the most important factors in promoting beautiful hair, as it fights off free radicals and protects the hair and scalp from DNA damage caused by environmental pollutants and everyday sun exposure. Nuts are a fabulous source of hair-nourishing Vitamin E, with walnuts, pine nuts and almonds offering some of the highest concentrations. Nuts are also high in the amino acid L-arginine, which is often used topically as a treatment for male baldness. Growing a healthy head of hair requires an abundant blood flow to the scalp, and L-arginine helps to improve this circulation by strengthening and increasing the flexibility of artery walls. Nuts rich in this powerful amino acid include cashews, almonds, pecans, hazelnuts and walnuts. I like to sprinkle nuts over my morning supercharged muesli and snack on a handful of them throughout the day. The other way that I boosted my nut intake was by replacing my regular milk with homemade nut milk. About a month after I did this my hair started to grow much thicker and looked healthier.

Sulphur is a dietary mineral that you may not hear about very often, but did you know that it's one of the most important nutrients in determining skin health? In fact, sulphur is the third most abundant mineral in the human body, and it's believed that a large proportion of the Western world is deficient in this vital mineral. Sulphur is required for the synthesis of collagen, which is well known for giving the skin structure, flexibility and strength. The insufficient production and breakdown of collagen is one of the primary contributors to premature skin aging. Increasing your intake of sulphur-rich foods is a wise investment into the quality of your skin, and you can find this complexion-perfecting mineral in egg yolks, grass-fed meats, chicken and fish. Rich plant sources of sulphur include onions, garlic and rocket (arugula), which also have a cleansing effect on the liver and the skin.

If weak, brittle nails are a problem for you, the last thing you need is another coating of nail-hardening solution. Solvents, glues, polishes and other conventional nail-care products contain a harmful cocktail of chemicals including formaldehyde, toluene and dibutyl phthalate (DBP) which are either suspected of, or known to cause allergies, endocrine disruption, reproductive issues, dermatological problems and respiratory illnesses. There is no time like the present to part with the polish, and look at the real causes of lifeless, fragile nails. These signs are often an indication of nutrient deficiency, and one of the nutrients closely related to nail health is silica. Silica is a mineral necessary for the strengthening and nourishing of the skin and nails, and has been regarded as one of nature's building blocks. Two of the foods that contain the highest concentration of silica are radishes and cucumbers. Red radishes contain the highest concentration of the mineral, but if you want to obtain it from your cucumber, then you must eat the skin. Always buy organic cucumbers, as the skin will not be tainted by pesticide residues and waxes. Jazz up your salads with these two ingredients and you'll be one step closer to diamond-strength nails, minus any nasty chemical side effects.

WRINKLE ACCELERATORS

Wrinkles are an inevitable part of life. When looking into some of the main factors contributing to aging, there are many simple dietary and lifestyle choices that you can make that will delay and even combat the presence of wrinkles, without breaking the bank, your skin or your health in the process.

A lack of elastin in the skin is one of the known trigger points in the development of wrinkles. Elastin is a structural protein that allows organs, including the skin, to stretch and recoil when movement takes place. A healthy presence of elastin in the skin means that it's free to move without creating creases and is more resilient, strong and flexible, and that it can maintain its original shape. One of the biggest elastin saboteurs is the sun. Sun damage causes a gradual destruction of elastin, resulting in a 'clumping up' of the skin and degradation of elasticity. Imagine an old, dry rubber band that's been left untouched in a drawer for many years: when you stretch it out, and it recoils, you can see the dry lines that have appeared. This is exactly the same effect that occurs with your skin in the absence of elastin.

The number one, obvious step to take to boost elastin is to avoid the sun and sun damage. However, avoiding sunlight altogether is not advised. Sunlight is a rich source of Vitamin D, a powerful anti-inflammatory which itself slows down the visible signs of aging. I would recommend staying out of strong midday rays and avoiding long hours in the sun. And choose a suncreen that is chemical-free to avoid damage to your skin.

There are particular foods that have been proven to prevent and fight against sun damage and which will help to keep the presence of your elastin fibres strong, regardless of a healthy exposure to sunlight. Incorporating sufficient protein into your diet is vital for maintaining healthy elastin levels in the skin, as it contains essential amino acids required for the production of elastin fibres. The most important amino acids for elastin production include lysine, glycine and proline, which can be found in grass-fed meats, beans, nuts, seeds and fish. There are plenty of recipes throughout the book that you'll find containing these wrinkle-wrangling ingredients.

Wild-caught salmon is a particularly powerful wrinkle-boxing food, not only because it is a source of elastin-building amino acids, but also because it's extremely high in omega-3 fatty acids, which help to lock moisture into skin cells, and offer further support for the maintenance and production of elastin fibres. I eat salmon a couple of times a week. Wild-caught salmon is known to be one of the highest forms of the super antioxidant astaxanthin, a carotenoid like lycopene. Carotenoid are crucial for plant photosynthesis and the protection of

plants and organisms from damage by light and oxygen, so it's no surprise that the presence of astaxanthin in wild salmon has been proven to reduce the sun damage caused to the skin by UV rays. Eating wild salmon regularly can help to maintain and boost elastin, and literally acts as an 'internal sunscreen', helping improve the appearance of fine lines and wrinkles, and increasing the tone, elasticity and moisture of the skin.

A lack of collagen is another factor that will prevent you from having a wrinkle-free complexion. Collagen is the main structural protein of our bodies, and similarly to elastin, acts as an enhancer of skin flexibility, elasticity and resilience. UV damage is a major cause in the degradation of collagen, however its presence will naturally diminish as you get older. As a person ages, collagen cells are less active and the skin becomes thinner and more prone to wrinkling. It is possible to delay and slow down this process through your diet.

Vitamin C is arguably one of the most important vitamins in the crusade against wrinkles. Some of the highest food sources of Vitamin C are papayas, strawberries, capsicums (peppers) and chillies, broccoli, brussels sprouts and citrus fruits. The best way to consume Vitamin C is in combination with Vitamin E, as the two protect each other from damage, and support one another in targeting sun damage and collagen and elastin degradation. Combining these fruits and vegetables with Vitamin E–rich chopped almonds or sunflower seeds in your salads or with breakfast is a great way to combine these power nutrients and reap the anti-wrinkle, collagen-boosting benefits they have to offer. Consuming Vitamins C and E–rich foods regularly will block the DNA damage caused by free radicals that can also lead to aging and wrinkles, as well as a range of age-related diseases including cancer, heart disease and arthritis.

By targeting wrinkles internally through whole foods, you are not only singling out the symptom of wrinkles, but are bringing health, vitality and longevity to your entire body in a good way.

ANTIOXIDANT-RICH FOODS

One theory of aging suggests that the role of oxyradicals and the antioxidant status of an individual is a major determinant in the rate of aging and age-related diseases. Oxyradicals, commonly known as free radicals, are active oxygen species that react adversely with the body's cells, resulting in a less efficient cell. In a normal situation, a balance exists among antioxidants, free radicals and biomolecules. But excess generation of free radicals may overwhelm natural cellular antioxidant defences, leading to oxidisation and contributing to cellular functional impairment and premature aging.

There is, however, no one single cause of aging. The role of oxyradicals is just one in the plethora of causes behind aging: a range of environmental and genetic factors such as geographical location, alcohol consumption, smoking, lifestyle and even gender all play a part in how we age. However, this doesn't detract from the importance of recognising that our antioxidant status *does* play a part in how we age at a cellular level. Countless studies reveal that free radicals can negatively alter the state of our cells, including our skin cells, over a lifetime, and that the presence of antioxidants will protect against these effects. It's also known that as we age, we are less able to deal with increased free radical activity; therefore it's paramount that our antioxidant status and our ability to minimise exposure to free radicals is addressed as we become older.

So how can you raise your antioxidant status? The most practical, safe, affordable and natural way to deal with the effects of pesky free radicals is through antioxidant-rich foods. Thankfully, Mother Nature has come to our rescue and all that we need can be found in delicious ingredients.

Vitamins A, C and E make up a serious power trio for encouraging tissue and cell growth, defending against the aging effects of sun damage, and environmental free radical damage, and encouraging the body to heal itself. This is particularly helpful for the skin, which continually sheds and replaces cells.

Vitamin A is made up of a broad group of related nutrients, and can be found in high quantities in sweet potatoes, carrots, spinach, kale, prawns and eggs. Vitamin A is required for healthy skin cell growth and development, and eating adequate quantities of foods containing Vitamin A will prevent the appearance of rough, dry and wrinkled skin.

Vitamin C acts as a powerful free radical scavenger, protecting DNA, cell membranes and collagen in the skin from the damage that comes with aging, and studies show that increasing your Vitamin C intake is associated with a better skin appearance with fewer wrinkles. Foods high in Vitamin C include papayas, capsicums (peppers), strawberries and broccoli. In fact, the humble broccoli is significantly higher in Vitamin C than an orange.

Vitamin E–rich foods include tocopherols and tocotrienols which are fat-soluble antioxidants known to protect the body against cancers, heart disease and premature aging. Vitamin E has actually been dubbed the 'master antioxidant' due to its immense power and ability to operate on a number of different levels in protecting against free radical–related aging. Its most important function seems to be in protecting cell membranes from oxidative damage. Boost your Vitamin E intake by regularly consuming walnuts and pecans, cold-pressed extra virgin olive oil and dark-green leafy vegetables.

Carotenoids are technically a precursor to, and subcategory of, Vitamin A. However this antioxidant is particularly powerful in the skin arena and so deserves mentioning on its own. Carotenoids include lycopene, beta-carotene and lutein, and are typically responsible for the red or orange pigments in fruits and vegetables. In recent years, carotenoid antioxidants have been recognised for their incredible anti-cancer and anti-aging compounds. Studies show that people with a lower

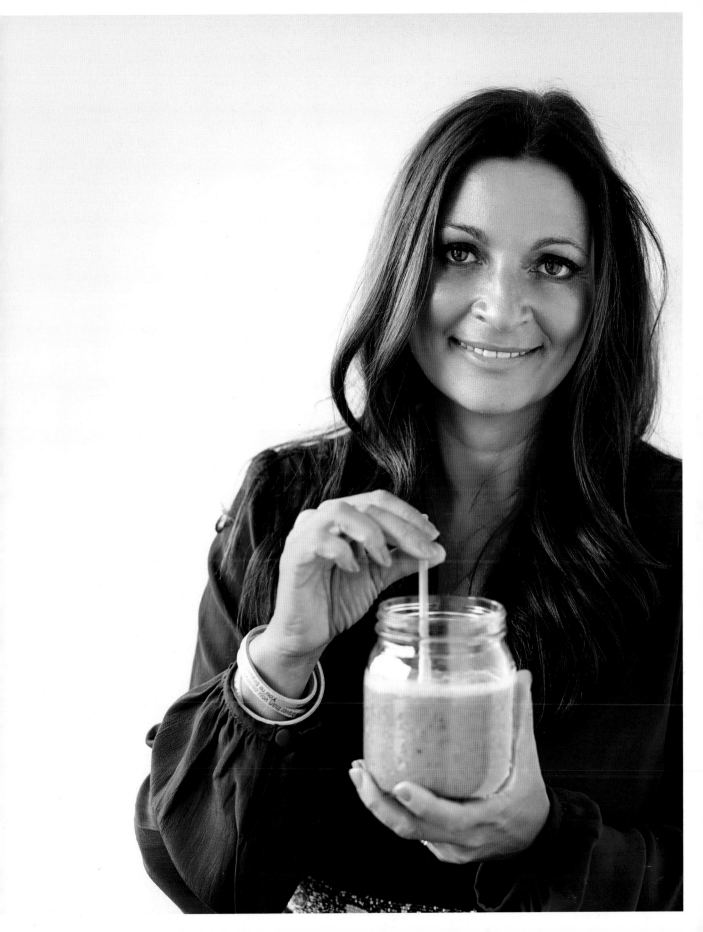

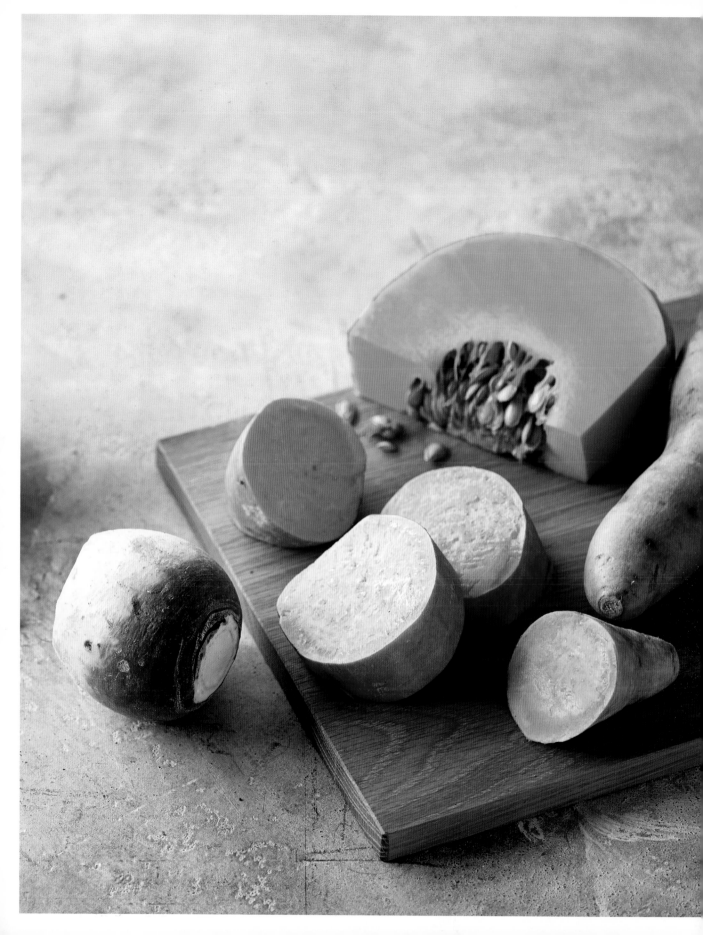

level of carotenoids in their skin are found to have deeper furrows and wrinkles than those with higher levels of carotenoids present. Foods high in carotenoids include carrots, apricots, tomatoes and sweet potatoes. Some green veggies are also surprisingly high in carotenoids, including English spinach, kale and collard greens. Consuming spices such as cayenne pepper and chilli powder is also a wonderful way to boost your carotenoid intake.

> For an antioxidant-rich snack place kale chips in the oven and then sprinkle them with a touch of chilli.

Polyphenols include resveratrol and flavonoid antioxidants, and have been recognised in several recent studies for their ability to prevent and slow oxidative aging on the body's cells, as well as a range of oxidation-related disorders. Green tea contains particular polyphenols known as catechins, which have a powerful anti-inflammatory effect on the body and may improve UV radiation–induced damage of the skin, as well as reducing inflammation, oxidative stress, and DNA damage to the skin. Research reveals that consuming the catechins in green tea improves skin hydration, transepidermal moisture loss, density and elasticity. Consuming polyphenol-rich foods has also been found to result in greater blood flow and oxygen supply to skin cells. Cinnamon, raw cacao, berries and red grape skins are also wonderful sources of polyphenol antioxidants that will help to protect your skin and keep your entire body free from oxidative stress.

VITAMIN- AND MINERAL- ABUNDANT FOODS

With the development of the modern pharmaceutical industry, there's been a gradual movement away from using whole foods as medicine and replacing them with isolated forms of nutrients and healing properties of foods which you can conveniently pop in synthetic pill form.

Nutraceuticals is now a particular area of widespread popularity and a broad concept that encompasses food-derived vitamins and minerals that contain specific medical effects. The word 'nutraceutical' was created from the words 'nutrition' and 'pharmaceutical', and covers a range of man-made, food-derived supplements and herbal products that claim to bring about a desired health result.

Nutraceuticals have even woven their way into the beauty and anti-aging industry, and can be found in both pill bottles and topical cosmetics. Popular groups of vitamins and minerals that feature in these products often include carotenoids, flavonoids, and nutrients with powerful antioxidant capacities including coenzyme Q10 and phytoestrogens, as well as probiotics and omega-3 fatty acids. While all of these individual nutrients have been scientifically proven to bring about health and beauty benefits, many scientists are beginning to suggest that a movement back towards food in its whole state is a smarter and cheaper approach to obtaining and effectively absorbing these potent nutrients.

Resveratrol is a naturally occurring polyphenol antioxidant that's found in particular plants. It is categorised as a phytoalexin, an antimicrobial compound that is produced by plants to protect them from rough environments like excessive UV light, infections and climate changes. Resveratrol has become an incredibly popular nutraceutical because of its scientifically proven ability to stimulate the production of a serum that slows down diseases and aging by speeding up the cells' energy production centres. Although resveratrol is found in red wine, it's not recommended to be consumed in abundance, as alcohol is a neurotoxin that can upset the body's delicate hormone balance as well as placing a toxic burden on the liver. The most potent food sources of resveratrol that you can consume safely include raw cacao products, red grape skins, mulberries and peanuts.

The nutraceuticals market offers these antioxidants as an antidote to free radical damage that causes aging, and there is much money to be made by selling these antioxidant supplements and topical concoctions. You'll notice that Vitamin C is often used in skincare and beauty supplements, promoted to enhance collagen production and prevent wrinkles. While science does back these antioxidant claims, I believe that it's more effective to keep the body topped up with Vitamin C from wholefoods, including citrus, strawberries, red and green chillies and capsicums (peppers), dark leafy greens, broccoli, watercress and kale, and herbs such as thyme and parsley. All of these foods not only boast Vitamin C, but also contain a range of other antioxidants that hold unique and complex benefits.

Coenzyme Q10 is possibly one of the most famous nutraceuticals on the supplement forefront. Browse the over-stocked supermarket beauty aisles and you'll notice that it's even more popularly used to market conventional 'anti-aging' creams and lotions. The science behind coenzyme Q10 justifies this phenomenon, with this age-busting nutrient being proven to prevent oxidative stress–induced cell death leading, to a reduction of facial wrinkles. When consumed, coenzyme Q10 offers incredible and measurable effects with respect to three major aging factors: oxidation, inflammation and methylation. It's also been proven to help with chronic illnesses including those of the cardiovascular system, neurological disorders and cancer. In its supplement form, coenzyme Q10 is very expensive, but can be found in high quantities naturally in wild-caught fish,

such as sardines, mackerel and tuna. If you're okay with organic offal, then beef, lamb or pork liver, kidney and heart are bursting with this wonder nutrient. Vegetables contain smaller amounts, but the highest in coenzyme Q10 include spinach and broccoli. Keep in mind that they must be consumed raw, fresh, unprocessed and organic wherever possible to ensure maximum nutrient levels are present.

Zinc deficiency is prevalent in the Western world and is is regularly supplemented in a synthetic form. It has excellent skin-healing properties. It is a mineral produced by the thymus gland. This gland is the site for T-cell production, and is large and robust during youth and adolescence but progressively shrinks after puberty. The presence of zinc is necessary for the healthy formation of DNA cell structures, lowering inflammation, fighting infection and preventing a range of age-related illnesses including cancer, diabetes and cardiovascular disease. In fact it is responsible for the triggering of over 100 differing internal enzymes required to help the body metabolise food. Zinc can be found in organic, grass-fed meats, poultry and seafood, especially oysters. Pepitas (pumpkin seeds) are also extremely high in this life-promoting mineral, and for maximum uptake, they should be eaten raw.

A lack of iron in diets can be attributed to brittle nails, so if yours are weak, spoon-shaped or thin, up your intake of iron by eating fresh green vegetables, nuts, seeds and lean red meat.

Increasing your Vitamin D levels can assist with inflammation. In a study conducted with 2000 women, those with higher Vitamin D levels were found to have less age-related changes and lower inflammatory markers. Food sources that contain high amounts of Vitamin D include fish, oysters and cod liver oil.

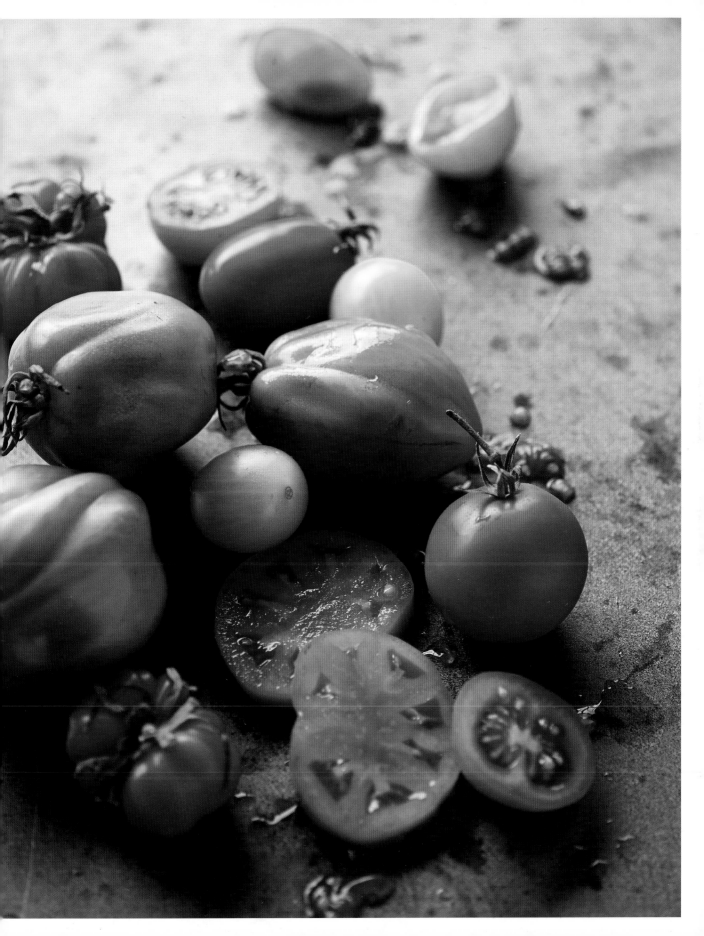

SHOPPING LIST

When you open your fridge do you see nothing but a few limp vegetables and a couple of old takeaway containers? Getting takeaway once in a while isn't a bad thing, but it's a lot smarter on your wallet and health to have a stocked fridge and pantry.

If you shop on a Saturday, you can use Sunday as a batch cooking day and then eat from the freezer through the week. Always check labels and look for the least processed, additive-free version of each food, making sure it's as close to its natural state as possible. The best meat to buy is grass-fed where your budget allows and the best seafood is wild caught. Look for seasonal organic fruits and vegetables where possible.

Shop smart with this extensive grocery list. There are dozens of tasty food options to help you get on the road to a beautifying diet. Copy it and take it on your next shopping trip.

VEGETABLES
Bok choy (pak choy)
Broccoli
Butternut pumpkin
  (squash)
Cabbage
Capsicum (pepper)
Carrots
Cauliflower
Celery
Cherry tomatoes
Cress
Cucumber
Eggplant (aubergine)
Garlic
Green beans
Kale
Lettuce greens
Onions
Parsnips
Peas
Pumpkin (winter
  squash)
Rocket (arugula)
Shallot
Silverbeet (Swiss chard)
Snow peas (mangetout)
Squash
Spinach leaves
Spring onions
Sprouts (all)
Swede (rutabaga)
Sweet potatoes
Tomatoes
Turnip
Watercress
Zucchini (courgette)

MEATS (PREFERABLY ORGANIC)
Beef
Lamb
Pork
Chicken
Duck
Turkey
Veal
Ham/Bacon
  (nitrate free)
Prosciutto

SEAFOOD
Salmon (wild caught)
Fresh fish
Anchovies
Prawns (shrimp)
Squid
Tuna
Sardines
Scallops
Sashimi
Sea vegetables

EGGS ORGANIC
Eggs

DAIRY (FULL FAT)
Organic butter
Organic cream
Goat's cheese
Sheep's cheese
Cow's cheese
Parmesan cheese
Plain yoghurt
  (no additives)

FATS AND OILS
Extra virgin olive oil
  (cold-pressed)
Coconut oil
  (extra virgin)
Seed & nut oils
Sesame oil

SEEDS, NUTS AND NUT BUTTERS

Hazelnut
Brazil
Macadamia
Pecan
Walnut
Almond
Pepitas (pumpkin seeds)
Chia seeds
Flaxseeds
Sesame seeds
Sunflower seeds
Poppy seeds
Pine nuts
Almond slivers
Tahini

BEANS AND LEGUMES

Cannellini
Lentils
Black
Pinto
Navy (haricot)
Split peas
Chickpeas

GRAINS, FLOURS AND BAKING

Almond flour
Coconut flour
Arrowroot flour
Arrowroot powder
Buckwheat groats,
  flour and pasta
Brown rice and brown
  rice noodles
White rice
Quinoa
Buckwheat
Spelt

Millet
Amaranth
Gluten-free
  self-raising flour
Golden flaxmeal
Baking powder
  (gluten- and
  additive-free)
Bicarbonate of soda
  (baking soda)
Coconut flakes
Desiccated coconut
Rice paper wrappers
Brown rice puffs
Cacao powder
Cacao nibs
Cacao butter
Coconut flakes
Alcohol-free
  vanilla extract
Vanilla beans

FRESH HERBS AND SPICES

Basil
Chives
Mint
Rosemary
Oregano
Cardamom
Coriander
  (cilantro)
Parsley
Sage
Thyme
Dill
Cumin
Ginger
Nutmeg
Cinnamon

CONDIMENTS AND SWEETENERS

Celtic sea salt
Fresh black pepper
Wheat-free tamari sauce
Apple cider vinegar
Stevia drops
Stevia powder
Xylitol
Coconut sugar
Rice malt syrup
Vegetable stock
  (sugar- and
  additive-free)
Tomato paste
  (concentrated purée)
Coconut aminos
Coconut nectar
Dijon mustard
Dulse flakes
Brown rice crackers

MILKS AND DRINKS

Nut milks
Rice milk
Full-fat organic milk
Coconut milk
Soda water

FRUITS

Apples
Bananas
Citrus
Avocados
Berries
  (fresh and frozen)

SEVEN-DAY BEAUTY MEAL PLAN

	BREAKFAST	LUNCH	DINNER	DESSERT
MONDAY	Warm Water with Lemon; Kale and Lemon Zest Omelette (page 66)	Wild Mushroom, Tomato and Spinach Frittata (page 146) with Sweet Potato, Celery and Apple Salad (page 143)	Chicken Casserole with Macadamia and Basil with Brown Rice (page 177)	Home-Style Apple Crumble (page 210)
TUESDAY	Warm Water with Lemon; Goat's Cheese and Raspberries on Chia and Flaxseed Loaf (page 72)	Carrot, Lemon and Fresh Mint Soup (page 121) with a slice of Mushroom and Almond Loaf (page 176)	Supercharged Lasagne with Steamed Green Beans (page 189)	Layered Quinoa Trifle (page 200)
WEDNESDAY	Blueberry Colada (page 56); Strawberry and Banana Breakfast Bake (page 70) with almond milk	Turmeric, Cauliflower and Almond Salad (page 136)	Moroccan Lamb Soup (page 114) with Sweet Potato Bread (page 220)	Raspberry-Studded Pumpkin Pie (page 194)
THURSDAY	Nutrient-Rich Green Juice (page 56); Almond and Apple Pancakes (page 76)	Crunchy Gado Gado (page 141)	Baked Wild Salmon with Parsley and Walnuts (page 169) with Seaweed and Sesame Salad (page 127)	Foolish Fudge Brownie (page 193)
FRIDAY	Warm Water with Lemon; Chia Seed Scramble on Spinach Loaf (page 77)	Keen-wah Burgers (page 160) with Turmeric and Rosemary Sweet Potato Fries (page 101)	Buckwheat Risotto with Spinach and Mushroom (page 186)	Berries with ACV and Cashew Nut Cream (page 204)
SATURDAY	Avocado and Spinach Smoothie (page 59)	Supercharged Omelette (page 66)	Fish and Vegetable Curry with brown rice (page 165)	Easy Sweet Potato Ice Cream (page 211)
SUNDAY	Crepes with Goat's Cheese and Wilted Baby Spinach (page 78)	Fish with Macadamia Salsa (page 158) and Red Cabbage and Apple Slaw with Tahini Dressing (page 128)	Lamb Pot Roast with Roasted Turnips and Steamed Broccoli (page 171)	Avocado and Chocolate Mousse (page 206)

*Beep beep. You have
a missed call. It's the
recipes calling to tell
you it's time to indulge
in luscious, health-
promoting food.*

Are you ready to eat yourself beautiful? Even if you're not ready to give up all of your indulgences just yet, why not try incorporating a few of the following nutra-gasmic, health-promoting recipes, loaded with vitamins and antioxidants, which will slow the clock with every mouthful.

You'll find time-rewinding nutritious drinks and smoothies, delicious and easy-to-make hunger-busting breakfasts and hearty soups and salads full of serious go power. If the main meal of the day is what you most look forward to, come in and indulge in dinners which will give you a glowing, golden hue inside and out and polish it off with a spoon-licking dessert. Enjoy your food adventures.

'Grow old along with me!
The best is yet to be.'
ROBERT BROWNING (1812-1889)

GUIDE TO ICONS
▲WF ▲DF ▲GF ▲SF ▲VG

If you're wondering what the at-a-glance icons next to the recipes are all about, here's a description so that you can find the recipes that best suit you.

▲**WF WHEAT FREE** Wheat is often found in products such as cereal beverages, breads and cereals, prepared mixtures such as pancakes and waffles, biscuits and crackers, salad dressings and sauces such as soy, luncheon meats, malted milk, modified starches, tinned soups and crumbed vegetable products. It's important to remember to scour labels for hidden ingredients. For some people, wheat is hard for their sensitive guts to digest and can cause allergic reactions. Common symptoms of a wheat allergy can include eczema, hives, asthma, hay fever, irritable bowel syndrome, tummy aches, bloated stomach, nausea, headaches, joint pain, depression, mood swings and tiredness. Wheat products can be replaced with buckwheat, rice, quinoa, tapioca and wheat-free flours.

▲**DF DAIRY FREE** A test for an allergy to dairy can be carried out by your doctor. These are skin-prick tests or blood allergen specific IgE (RAST) tests. The most effective way to test for a dairy allergy is to do an elimination. To avoid dairy in the supermarket look on labels for any food which contains cow's or goat's milk, cheese, butter, ghee, buttermilk, cream, crème fraîche, milk powder, whey, casein, caseinate and margarines which contain milk products. Substitutes for dairy milk include rice milk, nut and seed milks, oat milk and coconut milk.

▲**GF GLUTEN FREE** Gluten is a mixture of proteins found in grains such as wheat, rye, barley and oats. Some people can tolerate oats but the tricky bit is finding oats that haven't been contaminated by wheat or other grains during processing. Symptoms of gluten sensitivity can

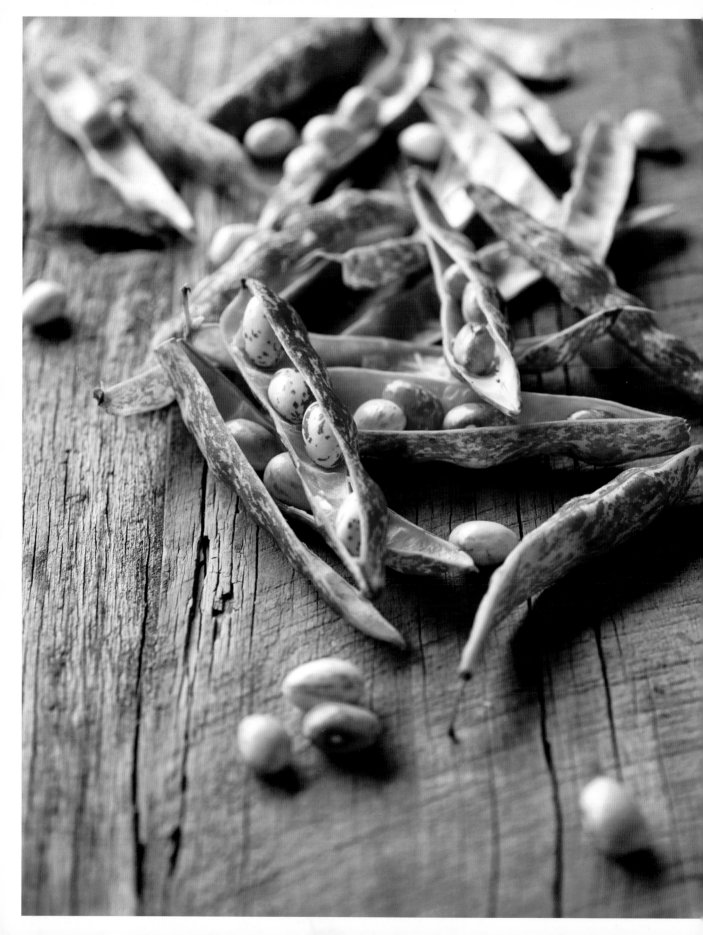

include gastrointestinal issues, skin problems, changes in weight, headaches and depression. Gluten sensitivity can make you feel ill or uncomfortable and can affect your mood and quality of life.

▲ **SF SUGAR FREE** Sugar is addictive and is everywhere, from muesli bars to yoghurt and even in frozen peas, sausages and tomato sauce (ketchup). Some of the worst offenders are between-meal sugary snacks or drinks which affect your appetite. Sugar can contribute to nutrient deficiencies and researchers have reported that a person with vitamin and mineral deficiencies such as magnesium, zinc, fatty acids and B group vitamins are more than likely to show symptoms of anxiety and depression. Some people have trouble digesting certain sugars that affect their digestion and internal gut flora, causing loose bowel actions or constipation and making them more prone to a build-up of bacteria in the gut and to yeast infections. Try putting nutrient-dense snacks ahead of sugar-filled snacks if you're looking for a quick fix. For the purposes of this book if a recipe contains fruit I have denoted that it is not sugar free so it won't contain the (SF) icon.

▲ **VG VEGETARIAN** These recipes contain no meat or eggs (though they may contain animal produce such as dairy, not suitable for vegans). If you are vegetarian, in order to ensure you are eating enough of the essential nutrients needed for optimum health, it is a good idea to include forms of protein, iron, Vitamins B12 and D and calcium in your diet. Good fats from non-meat sources are also very important. Eating a wide variety of real foods and not cutting out whole food groups unless absolutely necessary is a philosophy which works well for many people long-term.

'To eat is a necessity, but to eat intelligently is an art.'
FRANÇOIS DE LA ROCHEFOUCAULD
(1613-1680)

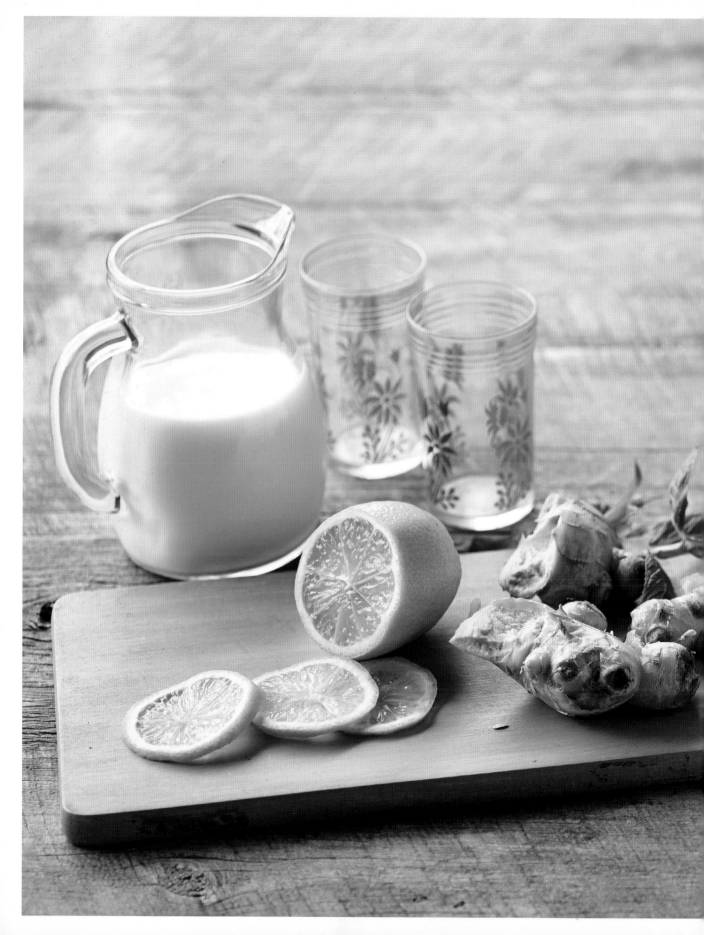

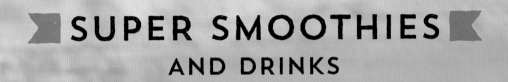

SUPER SMOOTHIES
AND DRINKS

For a ridiculously wholesome start to the day, stick these recipes onto your fridge door and whip up a vitamin-packed morning smoothie. Nightcappers, wind it down with an anti-inflammatory warming tea.

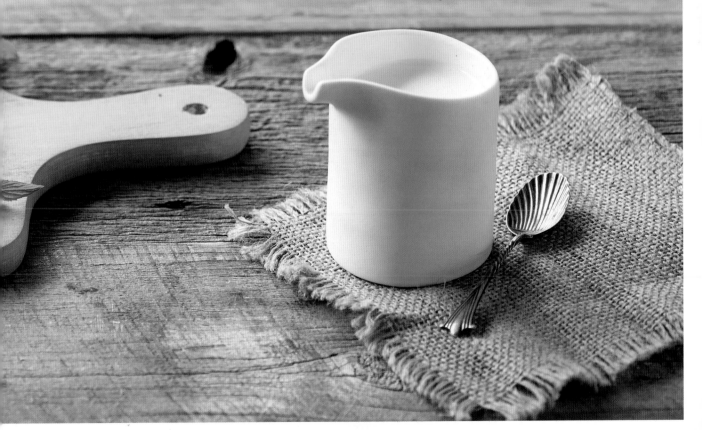

FOUNTAIN OF YOUTH

▲WF ▲DF ▲GF ▲VG   SERVES 1

Grapefruit has a high concentration of lycopene, a phytochemical that reduces the effects of free radicals. It will naturally boost your immune system, flush toxins, feed vital organs and cleanse you from the inside out. Drink this regularly for a healthier, glowing, iridescent skin and you'll be ready for your close-up.

1 grapefruit, peeled and quartered

4 strawberries, hulled and sliced

1/2 avocado, peeled, pitted and flesh cut into chunks

1 handful of parsley

1 handful of mint

4 ice cubes

250 ml (9 fl oz/1 cup) coconut water

Put all the ingredients into a blender and blend until smooth. For a thinner juice, add more coconut water.

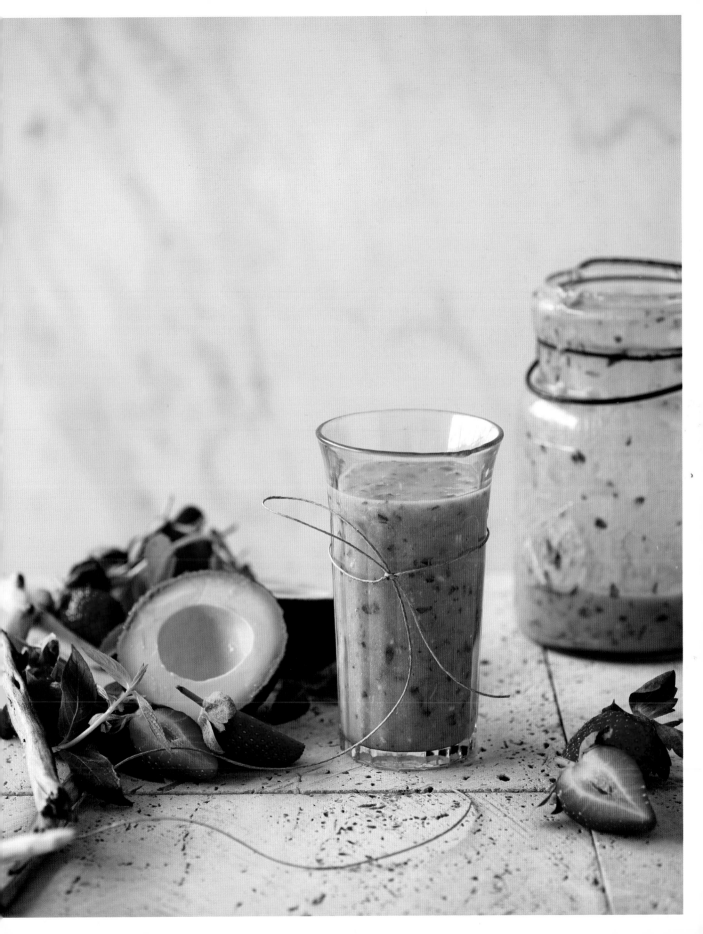

BLUEBERRY COLADA

▲WF ▲DF ▲GF ▲VG SERVES 2

Why not kick-start your morning with an on-the-go disease-preventing blueberry colada, bubbling with detoxifying antioxidants and packed with Vitamin C? The good fats in the nut butter and coconut will deliver an injection of nutrients directly into your body for maximum effect and the blueberries are the ultimate skin tonic.

155 g (5¹/₂ oz/1 cup) fresh blueberries (see note)

125 ml (4 fl oz/¹/₂ cup) additive-free coconut milk

125 ml (4 fl oz/¹/₂ cup) coconut water

40 g (1¹/₂ oz) nut butter

6 drops stevia liquid

1 teaspoon alcohol-free vanilla extract

1 teaspoon coconut flakes, to serve

Put all the ingredients, except the coconut flakes, in a blender and blend until smooth. Top with the coconut flakes and serve.

For a thinner smoothie, add more coconut water.

NOTE: If fresh blueberries aren't in season, use 125 g (4¹/₂ oz/1 cup) frozen berries instead.

NUTRIENT-RICH GREEN JUICE

▲WF ▲DF ▲GF ▲VG SERVES 1

Four good reasons to drink green juice:
★ *It's a major detoxifier and internal cleanser*
★ *It helps alkalise the body*
★ *It supports and strengthens the immune system*
★ *It provides energy*

2 kale leaves, washed and stems removed

1 bunch English spinach leaves

250 ml (9 fl oz/1 cup) coconut water

40 g (1¹/₂ oz/¹/₄ cup) fresh or frozen blueberries

1 teaspoon flaxseeds

1 teaspoon chia seeds

1 teaspoon spirulina powder

Put all the ingredients in a blender and whizz until smooth. It's that simple!

▶**SUPERCHARGED TIP**◀

If you fancy even more green goodness, pop in half an avocado.

THE KICK-START SHAKE

▲WF ▲DF ▲GF ▲VG   SERVES 2

This delicious protein-rich smoothie will kick-start your day with a mix of good fats and vitamins while being as smooth as silk on the stomach.

500 ml (17 fl oz/2 cups) almond milk (see note)

80 g (2³/4 oz/¹/2 cup) fresh or frozen blueberries

1 ripe banana

1 tablespoon coconut oil

1 tablespoon tahini

1 tablespoon ground flaxseeds

¹/2 teaspoon ground cinnamon

¹/4 teaspoon vanilla bean powder (or a dash of alcohol-free vanilla extract)

pinch of Celtic sea salt

Pop all the ingredients into a blender and blend until smooth and frothy.

NOTE: If you don't like almond milk, simply substitute the same quantity of your favourite nut milk.

►**HEALTH BENEFITS**◄

Along with their many other health benefits, coconut oil and flaxseeds are particularly stimulating for the digestive system.

BANANA, ALMOND AND FLAX SMOOTHIE

▲WF ▲DF ▲GF ▲VG   SERVES 1

For those on the run, warning, you'll become infatuated with this breakfast in a glass. It's the kind of fulfilling smoothie that will take you through to lunchtime and is bursting with vitamins, minerals and anti-inflammatory fats.

1 medium to large frozen banana, cut into chunks

20 g (³/4 oz) almond butter

1 tablespoon ground flaxseeds

170 ml (5¹/2 fl oz/²/3 cup) almond milk

6 drops stevia liquid

¹/2 teaspoon alcohol-free vanilla extract

Toss all the ingredients into a blender and blend until smooth.

►**SUPERCHARGED TIP**◄

Grind flaxseeds in a coffee grinder. Keep them refrigerated so they maintain freshness for longer.

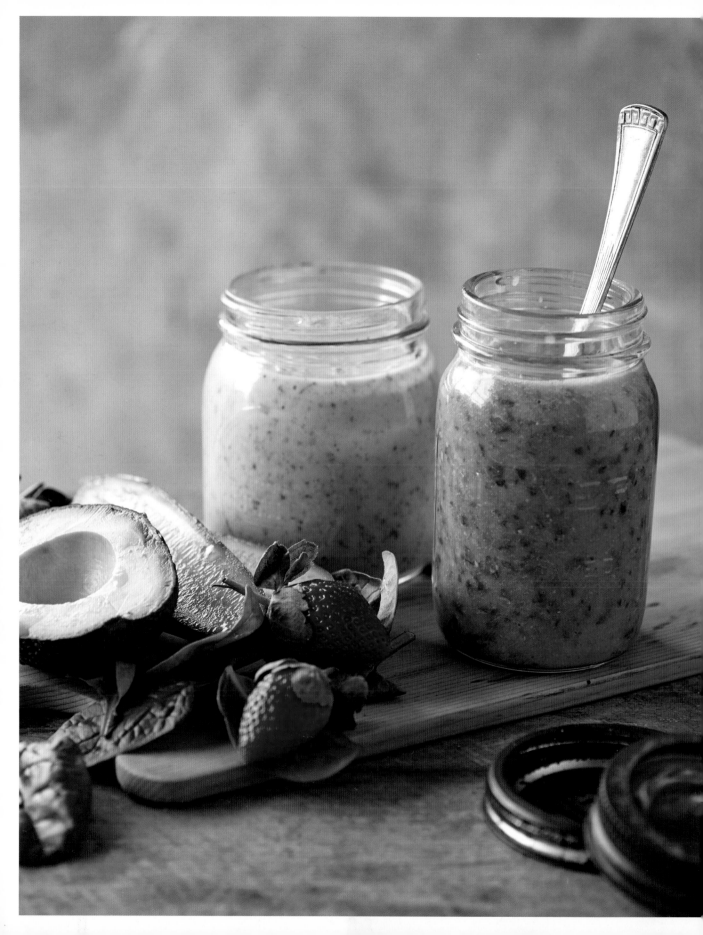

AVOCADO AND SPINACH SMOOTHIE

▲WF ▲DF ▲GF ▲SF ▲VG   SERVES 1

Avocado is a genuine beauty booster, and a great source of Vitamin E, enhancing the skin's vitality and luminosity. Its high Vitamin C content reduces skin inflammation, while avocado oil stimulates the production of collagen in the skin, to tone and improve its texture.

1/2 large avocado, peeled, pitted and flesh cut into chunks

1 bunch English spinach leaves

1 Lebanese (short) cucumber

250 ml (9 fl oz/1 cup) coconut water

125 ml (4 fl oz/1/2 cup) almond milk

Place all the ingredients in a powerful blender and whizz until smooth and creamy.

BEAUTY-BOOSTING SMOOTHIE

▲WF ▲GF ▲VG   SERVES 1

Needing to ramp up your beauty routine? Hey presto! For a quick and easy beauty boost, prettier hair, skin and nails, aim to down this a couple of times a week. The good news is it tastes as good as it makes you feel.

30 g (1 oz/1/4 cup) ground sunflower seeds and pepitas (pumpkin seeds)

1 ripe banana

250 ml (9 fl oz/1 cup) almond milk

6 ice cubes

130 g (41/2 oz/1/2 cup) sheep's milk yoghurt (optional)

6 strawberries, hulled

Put all the ingredients in a blender and blend until desired smoothness.

NOTE: For a dairy-free option, omit the yoghurt.

COMPLEXION BLEND TEA

▲WF ▲DF ▲GF ▲SF ▲VG   MAKES 2 CUPS

Skin is a mirror to internal health, and impeccable skin is not limited to 1930s silver screen goddesses or the genetically gifted. This tea will cleanse the bloodstream of impurities. The dandelion supports functioning of the liver, and a healthy liver is reflected through healthy and supple skin.

1 tablespoon dandelion root (or you can use instant ground powder or a dandelion tea bag)

1 tablespoon grated orange zest

2 cm (3/4 inch) piece of ginger, peeled and grated

1 tablespoon chopped mint leaves (optional)

stevia liquid, to taste

Add 500 ml (17 fl oz/2 cups) water to a small saucepan and add the dandelion root, orange zest, ginger and mint, if using. Bring to the boil and simmer for 5 minutes, stirring occasionally. Remove from the heat and strain through a sieve before serving. Add a few drops of stevia, to taste.

NOTE: If you're using a tea bag, prepare the tea in a pot, add the additional ingredients and steep for 5 minutes. If you prefer a milky dandelion tea, add a small amount of almond milk to the finished tea.

▶**HEALTH BENEFITS**◀

Dandelion is a source of potassium, sodium, calcium, phosphorus and iron. The leaves are a richer source of Vitamin A than carrots and contain some amounts of Vitamins B, C and D. The root contains bitter glycosides, tannins, triterpenes, sterols, volatile oil, choline, asparagine and inulin. Dandelion root can be purchased online or from your local health food store.

LATE-NIGHT ANTI-INFLAMMATORY WARMING TEA

▲WF ▲DF ▲GF ▲SF ▲VG   SERVES 1

I'm crazy for this tea. For a calming night's sleep, sip this slowly half an hour before bed – it's especially good at reducing bloating and water retention and you'll wake up feeling energised.

1 decaf tea bag

60 ml (2 fl oz/¼ cup) boiling water

250 ml (9 fl oz/1 cup) almond milk

½ teaspoon ground cloves

¼ teaspoon ground cardamom

½ teaspoon ground turmeric

¼ teaspoon ground cinnamon

¼ teaspoon freshly grated ginger

stevia liquid, to taste

Steep the tea bag in a mug of boiling water for 10 minutes.

Heat the almond milk in a small saucepan over medium heat for 2–3 minutes and stir in the spices. Remove from the heat and pour into the mug with the tea. Add a few drops of stevia, to taste, and enjoy warm.

GREEN TEA CHILLER

▲WF ▲DF ▲GF ▲SF ▲VG   SERVES 2

Not just a favourite on St Patrick's Day, or the drink of choice of supermodels, green tea chillers will smooth out the skin and promote a sag-free complexion.

9 ice cubes

6 drops stevia liquid

60 ml (2 fl oz/¼ cup) coconut water or milk

60 ml (2 fl oz/¼ cup) strongly brewed
  and chilled green tea, or decaf green tea

6 mint leaves

Place the ice in a blender, followed by the remaining ingredients. Blend until smooth.

Serve in a chilled glass.

▶SUPERCHARGED TIP◀

Don't rush out to the pharmacy to stock up on toxic lotions and potions: research shows that green tea is naturally rich in antioxidants, to protect the body from free radicals and accelerated aging. Note that green tea does contain caffeine.

CLEANSING TURMERIC AND GINGER TEA

▲WF ▲DF ▲GF ▲SF ▲VG   MAKES 1 CUP

Turmeric is not just a sunny bright spice to curry up dishes, it's also commonly used in traditional Ayurvedic and Unani medicine. You'll love this cleansing tea with its alkalising and detoxifying properties which provide powerful anti-inflammatory action. Turmeric is a superhero ingredient that helps to heal and prevent dry skin, slow aging, diminish wrinkles and improve skin's elasticity. Indian women use turmeric as a facial cleanser and exfoliant.

250 ml (9 fl oz/1 cup) almond or rice milk

2 teaspoons ground turmeric

1 teaspoon freshly grated ginger

stevia liquid, to taste

Add the almond milk to a small saucepan and heat gently until it reaches room temperature.

Add the turmeric and ginger to a mug. Pour a small amount of warm milk into the mug and stir to create a liquid paste, ensuring there are no lumps. Add the remaining milk and sweeten with a few drops of stevia.

▶SUPERCHARGED TIP◀

If you are using fresh turmeric, handle with care as it stains easily. If you do happen to turn your favourite garment yellow try squeezing on lemon juice or dab the spot with a little eucalyptus oil to remove the stain.

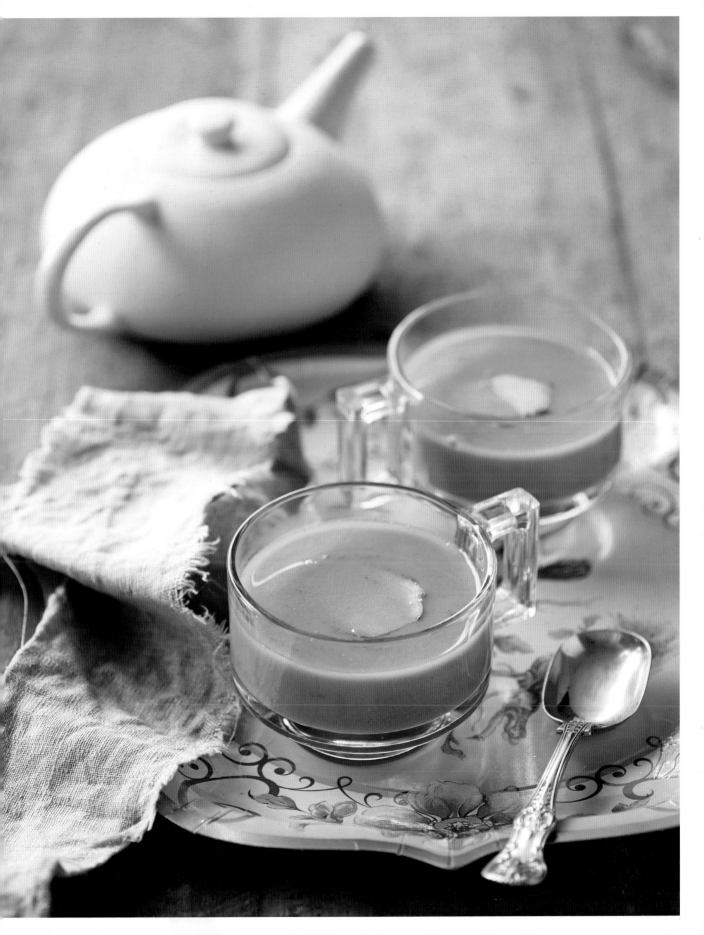

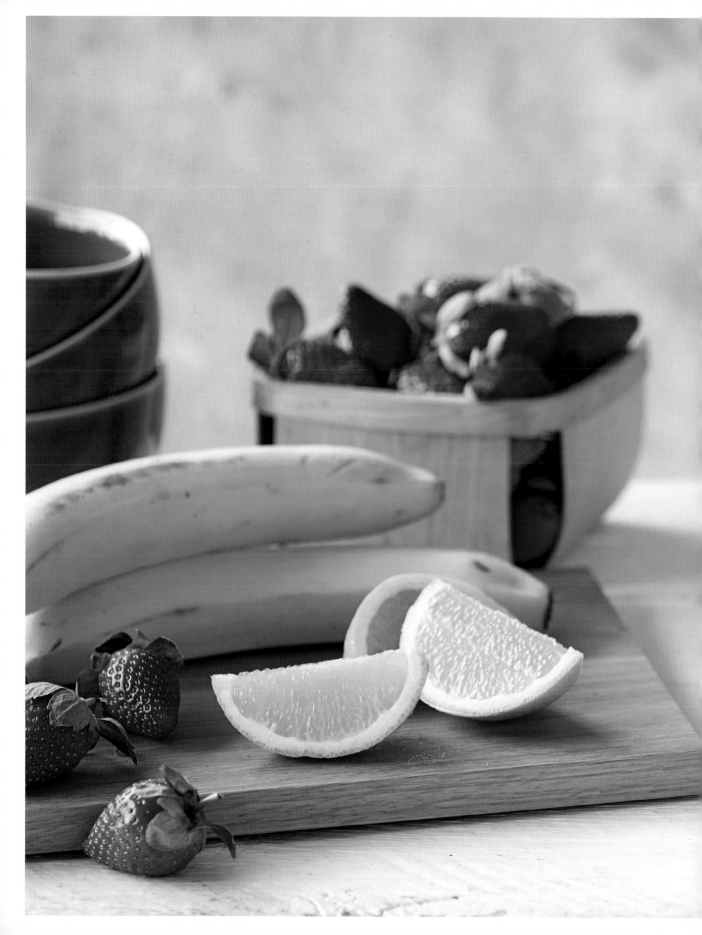

BREAKFAST

Move away from piggy products and builder's tea and be inspired by these delectable breakfast epiphanies.

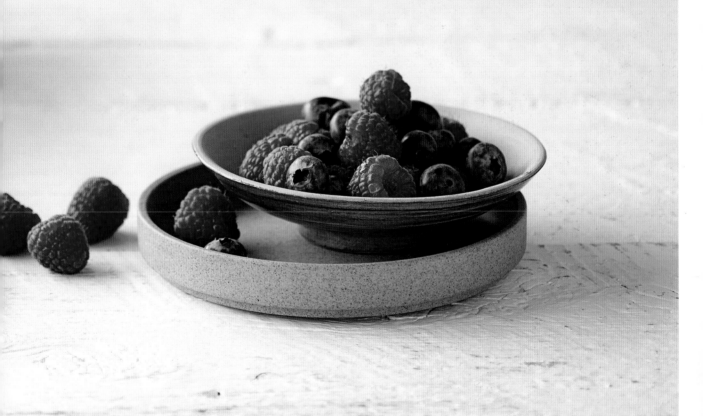

KALE AND LEMON ZEST OMELETTE

▲WF ▲DF ▲GF ▲SF   SERVES 1

The biotin found in eggs is fantastic for promoting luscious shiny hair, and the coconut oil and squeeze of lemon will help your body absorb and distribute beneficial iron from the kale.

1 tablespoon coconut oil

3 Tuscan kale leaves, washed, stems removed and shredded

1 tablespoon filtered water

1 tablespoon grated lemon zest

3 organic eggs, beaten

2 tablespoons finely chopped coriander (cilantro) leaves, plus extra to serve (optional)

lemon juice, to serve

Preheat the oven grill (broiler) to high.

Heat the coconut oil in a medium frying pan over medium heat and sauté the kale for a couple of minutes.

Add the water and lemon zest to the eggs, beat again and pour the egg mixture over the kale, giving the pan a swirl so the base is evenly coated.

Reduce the heat and scatter the coriander over the egg mixture. Cook for a minute or so, until the omelette is firm enough on the underside to be folded over. Tilt the pan away from you and use a spatula to gently lift and fold a third of the omelette on itself.

Transfer the omelette to the oven and cook for a further 5–10 minutes. Remove from the oven, transfer to a plate and top with a squeeze of lemon juice and the extra coriander, if using, and serve.

▶SUPERCHARGED TIP◀

Kale is a fantastic anti-inflammatory food. One cup of kale is filled with 10% of the recommended daily intake of omega-3 fatty acids, which will help your body fight against arthritis, asthma and autoimmune disorders. No wonder kale is now being called the queen green.

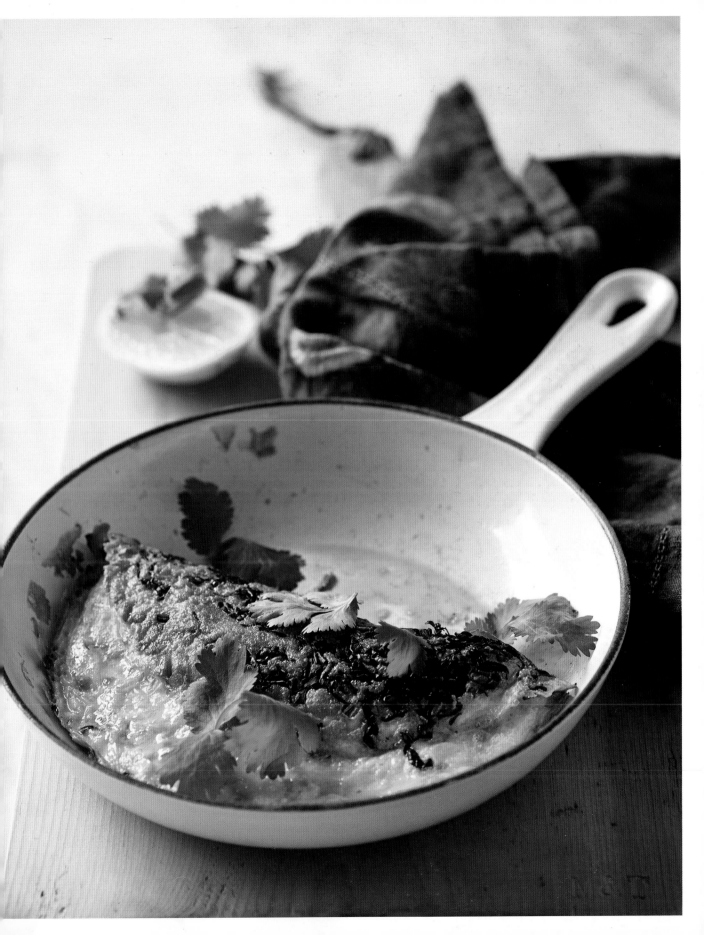

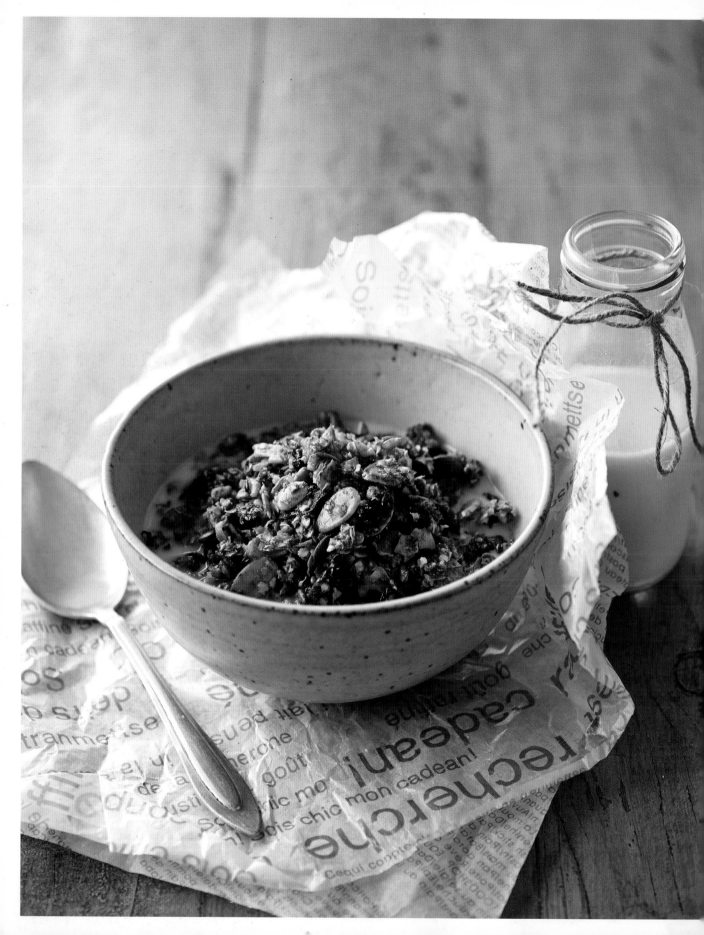

CRANBERRY AND WALNUT GRANOLA

▲WF ▲DF ▲GF ▲VG   SERVES 4

Tired of grinding your teeth on over-baked processed ready-made granola? It strikes me as odd that some packaged granolas have received health-food cult status. Store-bought varieties are usually full of sugar and brimming with bad fats. Whipping up a batch of this wholesome granola will bring out your inner earth mother (or father!), plus it moonlights as a cheeky nibble during the day. It's easy to swap out ingredients – as long as you stick to the basic mix you can make this granola your own.

300 g (10^{1}/$_{2}$ oz/1^{1}/$_{2}$ cups) **quinoa or brown rice flakes**

90 g (3^{1}/$_{4}$ oz/^{3}/$_{4}$ cup) **chopped walnuts**

75 g (2^{1}/$_{2}$ oz/^{1}/$_{2}$ cup) **dried cranberries**

3 tablespoons **sunflower seeds**

2 tablespoons **pepitas (pumpkin seeds)**

2 tablespoons **almond flakes**

1 tablespoon **flaxseeds**

^{1}/$_{2}$ teaspoon **ground cinnamon**

^{1}/$_{2}$ teaspoon **freshly grated nutmeg**

60 ml (2 fl oz/^{1}/$_{4}$ cup) **coconut oil**

60 ml (2 fl oz/^{1}/$_{4}$ cup) **rice malt syrup, or sweetener of your choice**

^{1}/$_{2}$ teaspoon **alcohol-free vanilla extract**

15 g (^{1}/$_{2}$ oz/^{1}/$_{4}$ cup) **coconut flakes**

almond milk, to serve

Preheat the oven to 180°C (350°F/Gas 4) and line a baking tray with baking paper.

Combine the quinoa, walnuts, cranberries, sunflower seeds, pepitas, almond flakes, flaxseeds, cinnamon and nutmeg in a bowl and mix well to combine.

Place the coconut oil in a saucepan over medium heat and heat until it has melted. Add the rice malt syrup and vanilla and stir for 30 seconds. Remove from the heat.

Pour the liquid mixture over the dry ingredients and stir well, ensuring the dry ingredients are coated thoroughly.

Transfer the granola to the baking tray in a single layer, then cook in the oven for 20 minutes, stirring frequently and breaking up any clumps that form. Remove from the oven, add the coconut flakes, and bake for a further 5 minutes.

Remove from the oven and cool.

To serve, place in a bowl and top with almond milk. It also tastes great on its own.

This granola keeps for 4 weeks in an airtight container in a cool dry place.

▶HEALTH BENEFITS◀

A quarter of a cup of walnuts can give you nearly 95% of your daily omega-3 requirements, and the huge amount of B vitamins they contain can not only help reduce stress, but keep your skin looking young, delaying the occurrence of fine lines and wrinkles.

STRAWBERRY AND BANANA BREAKFAST BAKE

▲WF ▲GF   SERVES 4

This is one of my favourite 'go to' recipes when I'm in the mood to start the day off with something warming, filling and delicious. It's perfect for any kind of company.

190 g (6³/4 oz/2 cups) gluten-free rolled oats (see note)

¹/2 teaspoon ground cinnamon

¹/2 teaspoon Celtic sea salt

140 g (5 oz/1 cup) chopped nuts of your choice

150 g (5¹/2 oz/1 cup) strawberries, hulled and chopped

560 ml (19¹/4 fl oz/2¹/4 cups) almond milk

60 ml (2 fl oz/¹/4 cup) rice malt syrup, or sweetener of your choice

1 organic egg

1 small apple, grated

1 teaspoon alcohol-free vanilla extract

1 ripe banana, sliced

1 tablespoon flaxseeds

2 tablespoons coconut flakes

milk of your choice, to serve

Preheat the oven to 190°C (375°F/Gas 5).

Place the oats, cinnamon, salt, half the nuts and half the strawberries in a bowl.

In a jug, whisk the almond milk, rice malt syrup, egg, apple and vanilla together.

Transfer the oat mixture to a 20 x 20 x 5 cm (8 x 8 x 2 inch) ovenproof tin. Scatter the remaining strawberries and nuts and the banana on top. Pour over the almond milk and egg mixture, letting it filter through the oats.

Bake in the oven for 20 minutes, or until golden brown.

Remove from the oven and sprinkle with the flaxseeds and coconut flakes.

Serve hot in a bowl and pour over milk to taste.

This will keep for 2–3 days in an airtight container in the fridge.

NOTE: You can also use 400 g (14 oz/2 cups) of quinoa or brown rice flakes instead of gluten-free oats. This is also dairy-free, if served with nut milk.

▶HEALTH BENEFITS◀

Strawberries contain biotin, which helps build strong hair and nails, and the antioxidant ellagic acid, which protects the elastic fibres in our skin to help prevent sagging. The phenols in strawberries also fight against many inflammatory disorders.

QUIRKY QUINOA MUFFINS

▲WF ▲GF ▲SF   MAKES 12 MUFFINS

These melt-in-your-mouth muffins are a great way to use leftover quinoa. They're the perfect lunchbox snack.

200 g (7 oz/1 cup) quinoa, rinsed

2 organic eggs

1 brown onion, finely chopped

200 g (7 oz) goat's cheese or grated full-fat cheddar cheese

1/2 cup roughly chopped coriander (cilantro) leaves

45 g (1 1/2 oz/1/3 cup) cherry tomatoes, diced

1/2 teaspoon Celtic sea salt

1/2 teaspoon freshly ground black pepper

Preheat the oven to 175°C (345°F/Gas 3–4) and line a 12-hole 60 ml (2½ fl oz/1/3 cup) muffin tin with paper liners.

Cook the quinoa according to the packet instructions.

Combine the cooked quinoa with all the other ingredients in a large bowl. Divide the mixture among the muffin holes and flatten off the top of each muffin with a spatula.

Bake for 20 minutes, or until golden brown. Remove from the oven and set aside on a wire rack to cool for 15 minutes.

These will keep in an airtight container in the fridge for 4 days.

▶HEALTH BENEFITS◀

Full of protein, these well-rounded muffins are a great energy-boosting breakfast and especially delicious when served warm. The cherry tomatoes contain the circulation booster lycopene and Vitamin C, which helps to keep the skin firm by aiding collagen production.

GOAT'S CHEESE AND RASPBERRIES ON CHIA AND FLAXSEED LOAF

▲WF ▲GF   SERVES 2

Chia seeds are the beauty buzz-word of the moment and a tiny but mighty way to stock up on omega-3s. If you don't feel like cereal then this is a speedy and yummy alternative. Use any berries that are in season. If you're avoiding dairy then nut butter is a worthy alternative.

2 slices chia and flaxseed loaf (see page 222)

100 g (3¹/₂ oz/¹/₂ cup) fresh goat's cheese, at room temperature

2 teaspoons sheep's milk yoghurt

60 g (2¹/₄ oz/¹/₂ cup) fresh raspberries, slightly mashed with a fork

Toast the bread.

Meanwhile, place the goat's cheese and yoghurt in a small bowl and mash with a fork until combined. Spread the mixture over the toast and top with a single layer of raspberries.

▶SUPERCHARGED TIP◀

Did you know that goat's milk contains 27% more of the antioxidant selenium than regular cow's milk? It's easier to digest and some people who are lactose intolerant can tolerate goat's cheese. The levels of lactose can be similar, but the fat molecules in goat's cheese are shorter, making them more digestible.

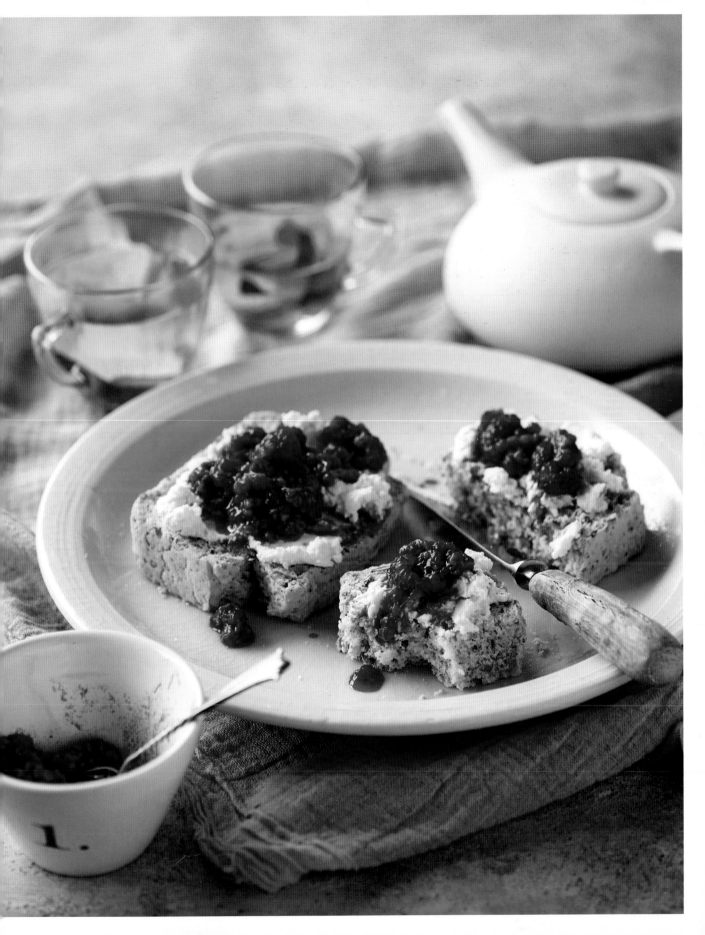

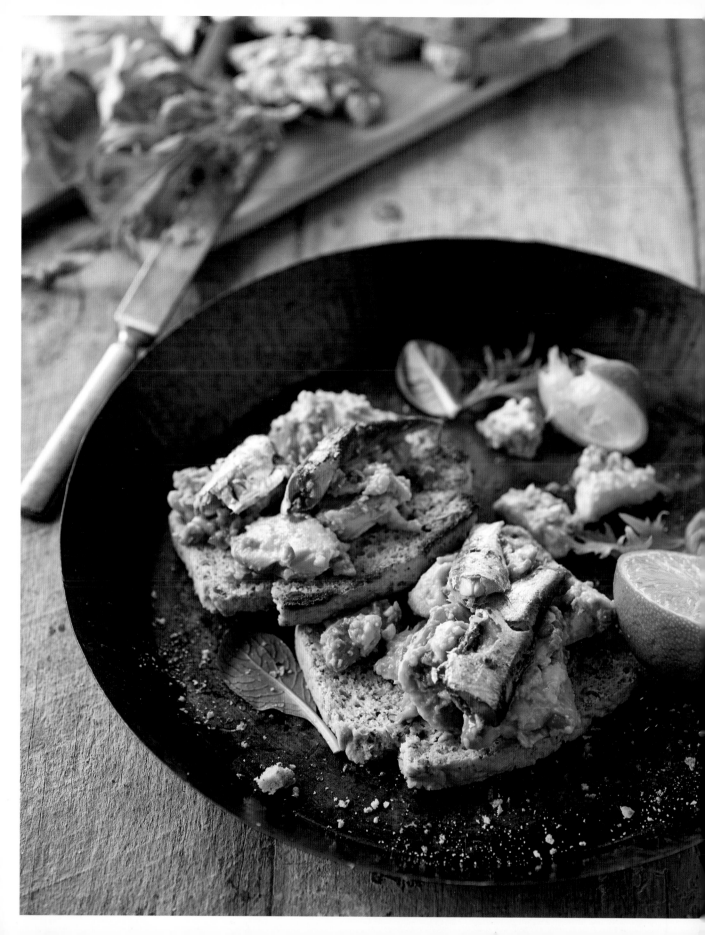

SARDINES WITH AVOCADO

▲WF ▲DF ▲GF ▲SF   SERVES 1

Sardines are one of the most powerful beauty boosters and their omega-3 content helps you avoid new wrinkles. Omega-3s are brilliant at oxygenating your skin tissue, revitalising and improving your skin tone and giving you a healthy glow.

1/2 avocado, peeled and stone removed

1 tablespoon freshly squeezed lime juice

1 teaspoon chopped red chilli (optional)

pinch of Celtic sea salt

freshly ground black pepper

1–2 slices Gluten-Free Bread (see page 218), or Chia and Flaxseed Loaf (see page 222)

1 small handful of rocket (arugula) leaves

120 g (4¼ oz) tin sardines, smashed

extra virgin olive oil, for drizzling

Place the avocado, lime juice, chilli, if using, salt and pepper in a bowl and mash together with a fork.

Toast one or two slices of your favourite gluten-free bread.

Spread the avocado mixture over the toast and top with the rocket and smashed sardines.

Drizzle with olive oil and serve with the lime wedges on the side.

▶HEALTH BENEFITS◀

The most intriguing benefit of sardines is that they help to slow the aging process. They are rich in the vital coenzyme Q10, which promotes a healthy immune system, restores vitality and is a potent antioxidant. The omega-3 oils in sardines benefit the circulatory system, have anti-inflammatory properties and hydrate the skin.

ALMOND AND APPLE PANCAKES

▲WF ▲GF   MAKES 8–10 PANCAKES

These fluffy breakfast delights are really lovely. The only real work involved in this recipe is grating the apple and a spot of whisking. They go down a treat with chai tea.

3 organic eggs

200 g (7 oz/2 cups) almond meal

170 ml (5¹/₂ fl oz/²/₃ cup) almond milk

1 small apple, grated

¹/₂ teaspoon alcohol-free vanilla extract

1 teaspoon ground cinnamon

pinch of Celtic sea salt

40 g (1¹/₂ oz) unsalted butter

stevia powder, to serve

In a large jug, whisk the eggs. Mix in the almond meal and milk, apple, vanilla, cinnamon and sea salt. Leave for 10 minutes to settle.

Add the butter to a large frying pan and place over medium–high heat until glistening.

Making several pancakes at a time, spoon the batter into the pan in 60 ml (2 fl oz/¹/₄ cup) quantities. Cook for about 2–3 minutes, or until the batter has set and is bubbling, then carefully flip the pancakes and cook them on the other side for a minute or two, or until browned to your taste.

Remove from the pan and keep warm while you cook the rest. Repeat with the remaining butter and batter until all the batter is cooked.

Serve warm, sprinkled with stevia powder.

CHIA SEED SCRAMBLE

▲WF ▲GF ▲SF   SERVES 2

Been up all night partying? Mercifully, here's a quick dish to unscramble the brain and give you an injection of protein. Chia seeds were a major staple in the diets of the Aztecs and Mayans. They were carried on long journeys by Aztec warriors and used to enhance their strength and endurance.

4 organic eggs

2 teaspoons almond milk

2 tablespoons chia seeds

20 g (3/4 oz) unsalted butter

2 garlic cloves, minced

1 brown onion, chopped

40 g (1 1/2 oz/1/4 cup) chopped red and yellow capsicum (pepper)

1 large handful of baby English spinach leaves

chopped coriander (cilantro) leaves, to garnish

Whisk the eggs and almond milk together in a bowl. Drop in the chia seeds and let it sit for about 15 minutes – the mixture should thicken up as the chia seeds expand.

Heat the butter in a medium frying pan over medium heat and sauté the garlic and onion until translucent. Add the capsicum and cook for about 3 minutes. Pour in the egg mixture and stir with a fork until it is almost set. Add the spinach and cook for about 1 minute or until the leaves have wilted.

Top with the coriander and serve.

▶HEALTH BENEFITS◀

Chia seeds are packed to the nines with antioxidants and omega-3 fats. They have the highest omega-3 content of any plant-based source, including flaxseeds.

CREPES WITH GOAT'S CHEESE AND WILTED BABY SPINACH

▲WF ▲GF ▲SF   SERVES 4

Flour power is alive and well. Bring these to the table and you'll be crowned the queen (or king) of the breakfast table.

60 g (2¼ oz) unsalted butter, melted

1 large handful of baby English spinach leaves, to serve

120 g (4¼ oz/1 cup) tapioca flour

250 ml (9 fl oz/1 cup) additive-free coconut milk

1 organic egg

pinch of Celtic sea salt

120 g (4¼ oz/1 cup) goat's cheese, to serve

Heat 1 tablespoon of the butter in a frying pan over medium heat and add the spinach leaves. Cook for 1 minute, or until they have wilted. Remove from the pan and set aside.

Put the flour, coconut milk, egg and salt into a medium bowl and mix well to combine.

Heat the remaining butter in a frying pan over medium heat. Pour in a quarter of the crepe mixture and swirl around so it covers the base of the pan. Cook for 2–3 minutes, then carefully flip the crepe and brown the other side. Remove from the pan and keep warm.

Repeat with the remaining mixture.

To serve, top the crepes with the goat's cheese and spinach.

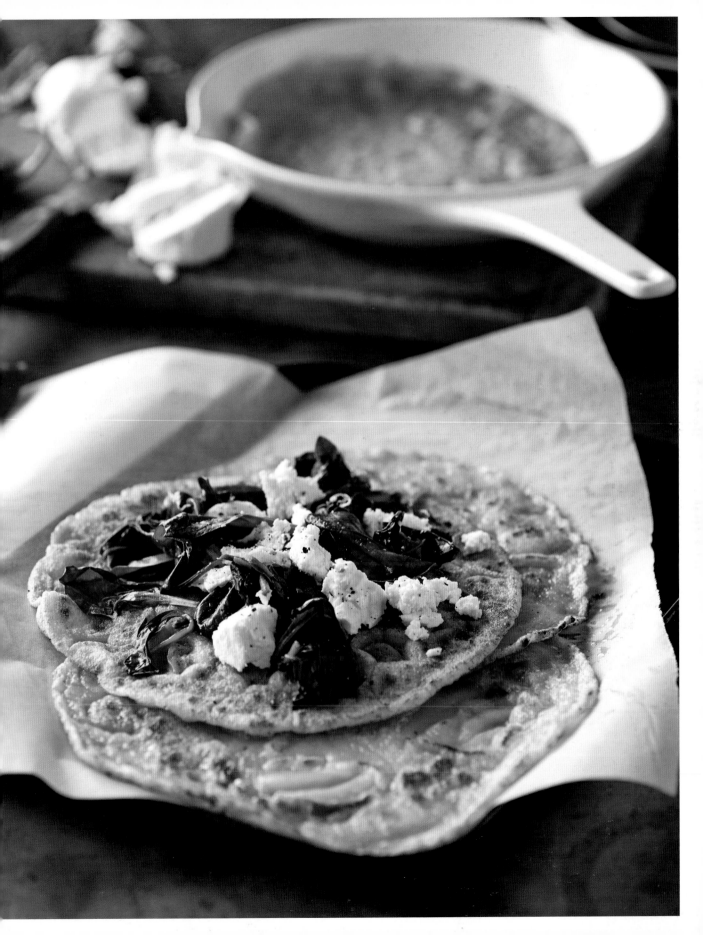

BLACKBERRY AND FLAXSEED PANCAKES

▲WF ▲GF　　　SERVES 2

These phenomenal pancakes are simply a joy to whip up. Blackberries and flaxseeds are the ultimate duo. Enjoy them late for breakfast on a lazy Saturday morning with the papers.

70 g (2¹/₂ oz/²/₃ cup) almond meal

2 tablespoons ground flax meal

1 tablespoon gluten-free baking powder

1 organic egg

6 drops stevia liquid

250 ml (9 fl oz/1 cup) almond milk

coconut oil, for pan-frying

65 g (2¹/₄ oz/¹/₂ cup) fresh blackberries
  (see note)

Greek-style yoghurt, to serve (optional)

In a mixing bowl, combine the almond meal, flax meal and baking powder. Add the egg, stevia and almond milk.

Add a light coating of coconut oil to a frying pan and place over medium–high heat. Gently ladle one-eighth of the batter into the pan and sprinkle some blackberries over the top.

When the pancake starts to bubble, gently flip it over and cook the other side. Continue to cook for 2–3 minutes, or until the pancake is set.

Remove from the pan and place on a waiting plate to keep warm while you make the remaining pancakes.

Repeat with the remaining batter and blackberries. Serve warm with Greek-style yoghurt, if desired.

NOTE: If blackberries aren't in season, you can substitute any other berries. If you don't serve this with yoghurt, it is also dairy-free.

▶HEALTH BENEFITS◀

Flaxseeds do more than boost the fibre content of a meal, they also supply a good dosage of essential fatty acids and they're colon friendly too.

ORANGE AND CRANBERRY BREAKFAST MUFFINS

▲WF ▲GF   MAKES 6 MUFFINS

A delicious, zesty and light muffin recipe that's short on sugar and big on taste. Score!

75 g (2½ oz/½ cup) coconut flour

1 teaspoon gluten-free baking powder

½ teaspoon bicarbonate of soda
  (baking soda)

1 teaspoon stevia powder, or sweetener
  of your choice

4 organic eggs

2 tablespoons freshly squeezed orange juice

75 g (2½ oz/½ cup) dried cranberries

1 tablespoon grated orange zest

1 teaspoon alcohol-free vanilla or
  orange extract

60 g (2 oz) unsalted butter, melted

125 ml (4 fl oz/½ cup) additive-free
  coconut milk

Preheat the oven to 180°C (350°F/Gas 4). Line a 6-hole 250 ml (9 fl oz/1 cup) muffin tin with paper liners.

Combine the coconut flour, baking powder, bicarbonate of soda and stevia powder in a bowl.

In a separate large bowl, mix the eggs, orange juice, cranberries, vanilla or orange extract, butter and coconut milk. Add the dry ingredients and combine well.

Pour the batter into the muffin holes and fill each liner to about three-quarters full.

Bake in the oven on the middle shelf for 15–20 minutes, or until a skewer inserted into the middle of a muffin comes out clean.

Remove from the oven and transfer to a wire rack to cool.

These will keep in an airtight container for 5 days.

▶SUPERCHARGED TIP◀

Coconut flour recipes typically call for more eggs due to the flour absorbing more moisture and soaking up liquids. If you are egg-free, substitute with ground flaxseed or chia seed and water; or arrowroot and tapioca starch.

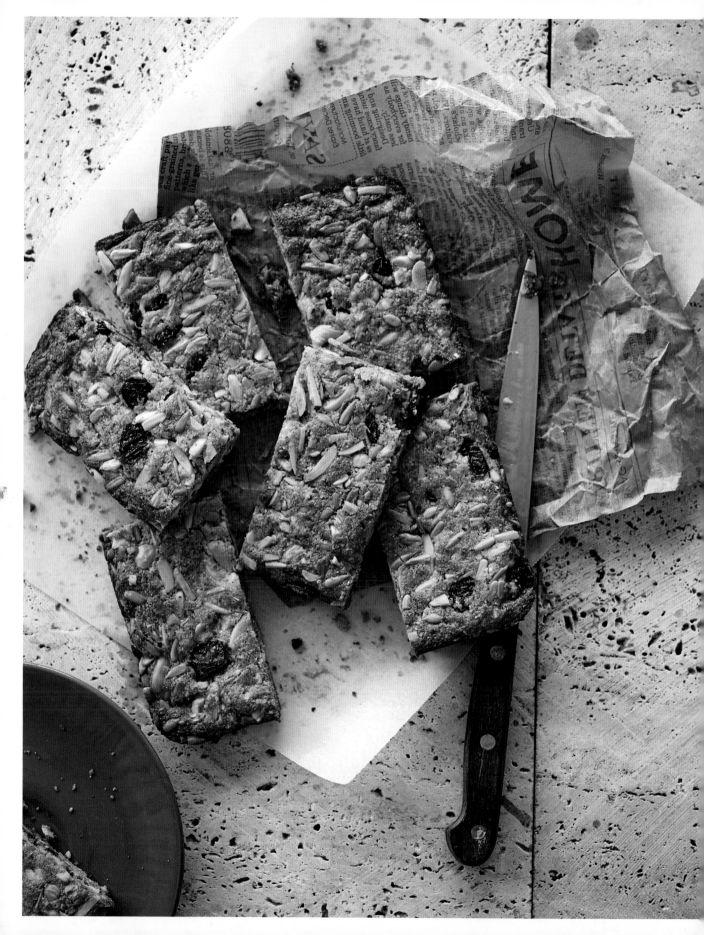

SUPERCHARGED BREAKFAST BARS WITH FSA

▲ WF ▲ GF   MAKES 8 BARS

Craving a morning energy boost? My breakfast bars are off the scale and a wonderfully safe port of call amid the storm of clichéd healthy breakfast bar options on the market. Plus they're bursting with skin-saving omega-3s.

unsalted butter, for greasing

125 g (4¹/₂ oz/1¹/₄ cups) almond meal

pinch of Celtic sea salt

¹/₄ teaspoon bicarbonate of soda (baking soda)

60 ml (2 fl oz/¹/₄ cup) coconut oil

60 ml (2 fl oz/¹/₄ cup) rice malt syrup, or sweetener of your choice

1 teaspoon alcohol-free vanilla extract

40 g (1¹/₂ oz/¹/₄ cup) cashews, crushed

160 g (5¹/₂ oz/1¹/₄ cups) combined flaxseeds, sunflower seeds and slivered almonds (FSA)

40 g (1¹/₂ oz/¹/₄ cup) dried cranberries (optional)

Preheat the oven to 175°C (345°F/Gas 3–4). Grease a 20 x 20 x 5 cm (8 x 8 x 2 inch) square ovenproof tin.

Mix the almond meal, salt and bicarbonate of soda together in a bowl.

In a separate bowl, combine the coconut oil, rice malt syrup and vanilla. Add the almond meal mixture, and mix in the nuts, seeds and cranberries, if using.

Wet your hands and then transfer the mixture to the tin, using your hands to press down firmly on the mixture.

Transfer to the oven and bake for 15–20 minutes.

Remove from the oven, transfer to a wire rack and cool before dividing into 8 bars and serving.

These will keep in an airtight container for 7–10 days.

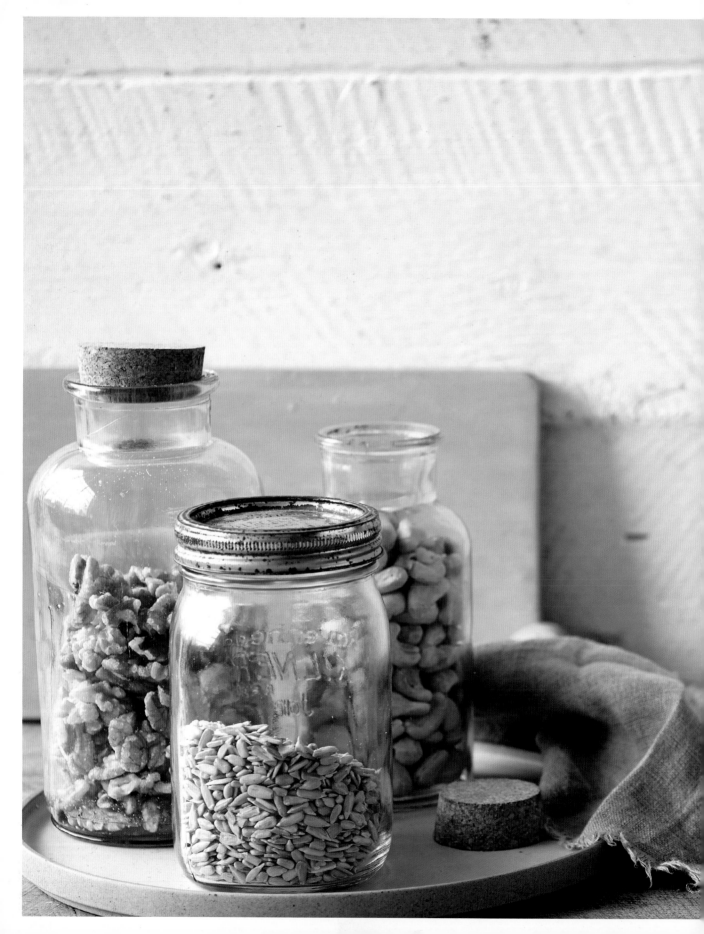

SNACKS, SIDES
AND BASICS

From flax crackers to seanuts, and stuffed mushrooms with pistachio to broccolini with garlic and chilli, get a load of these über healthy emergency snacks and sides. Add a bunch of delectable dressings and basics and spoon your way into every occasion. Go Vietnamese with a delicious Asian-style dressing or take your guests on a Moroccan adventure. Feeling saucy? Perk up salads with anti-inflammatory omega-3 mayo and discover your inner green goddess (or god) with a greenhouse spinach dip.

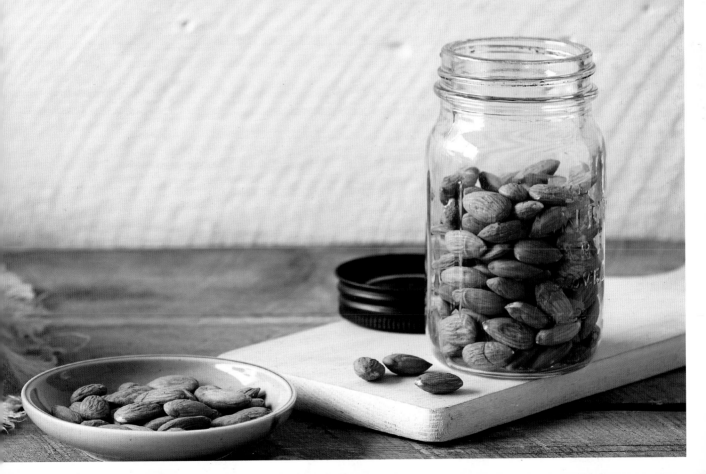

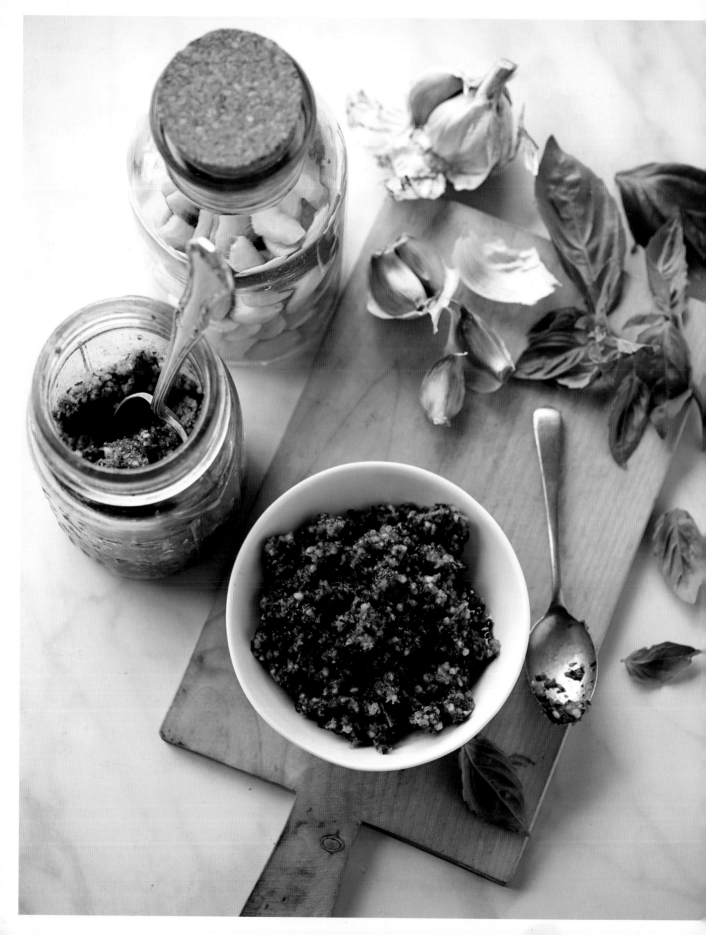

ALMOND PESTO

▲WF ▲DF ▲GF ▲SF ▲VG   MAKES 1 CUP

The addition of pesto makes otherwise mundane meals taste positively gourmet. Eat it alone or in combination with other dishes. You'll never buy another supermarket dip again. For variation, you can substitute the blanched almonds with sunflower or pepitas (pumpkin seeds).

160 g (5½ oz/1 cup) blanched almonds

2 garlic cloves, peeled

2 large handfuls of basil leaves

80 ml (2½ fl oz/⅓ cup) extra virgin olive oil

1 tablespoon freshly squeezed lemon juice

2 tablespoons nutritional yeast flakes

small pinch of Celtic sea salt

Place the almonds in a food processor and whizz until fine. Add the garlic and pulse, then add the basil and whizz again. With the motor running, slowly drizzle in the olive oil until you have the desired consistency, then add the lemon juice, yeast flakes and sea salt.

The pesto will keep in an airtight container in the fridge for a week and can be refreshed with an extra splash of olive oil.

NOTE: If it's looking dry, add more olive oil as required.

▶SUPERCHARGED TIP◀

This is delicious as a pizza topping, or give it a try on spiralised zoodles (zucchini noodles) pan-fried in garlic. (See page 155 for zoodle recipe.)

CANNELLINI BEAN AND WALNUT PÂTÉ

▲WF ▲DF ▲GF ▲SF ▲VG　　MAKES 1 CUP

Vegetarians be warned, this creamy uniquely flavoured savoury pâté is really hard to pick fault with and tastes delicious on seeded crackers. Store it in your fridge and serve it as a sandwich filling or all-round dip.

400 g (14 oz) tin cannellini beans, rinsed and drained

115 g (4 oz/1 cup) walnuts

1 garlic clove, peeled

1 tablespoon freshly squeezed lemon juice

1 tablespoon wheat-free tamari

1 1/2 tablespoons apple cider vinegar

1 1/2 teaspoons dried thyme

1/2 teaspoon freshly ground black pepper

1 teaspoon chopped rosemary leaves

Celtic sea salt, to taste

1 teaspoon grated lime zest

Put all the ingredients in a food processor and pulse until smooth.

Pour into an airtight container and put in the fridge to chill before serving.

This pâté will keep in an airtight container for 4–5 days in the fridge.

▰HEALTH BENEFITS▰

Walnuts contain healthy omega-3 fats to strengthen the membranes of your skin cells, kicking out toxins and locking in moisture to keep skin hydrated, plumped and glowing.

GREENHOUSE SPINACH DIP

▲WF ▲DF ▲GF ▲SF ▲VG　　MAKES 1 CUP

Six ingredients and you have a yummy dip in less than six minutes for when unexpected guests drop by. If you don't have fresh spinach, use thawed frozen spinach. Don't forget to squeeze out the excess water before using.

4 bunches English spinach leaves

1 large avocado, peeled and stone removed

1/2 red onion, roughly chopped

2 garlic cloves, peeled

large pinch of Celtic sea salt

juice of 1 lemon

Place all the ingredients in a food processor and process until creamy.

This dip will keep in the fridge for 5 days in an airtight container.

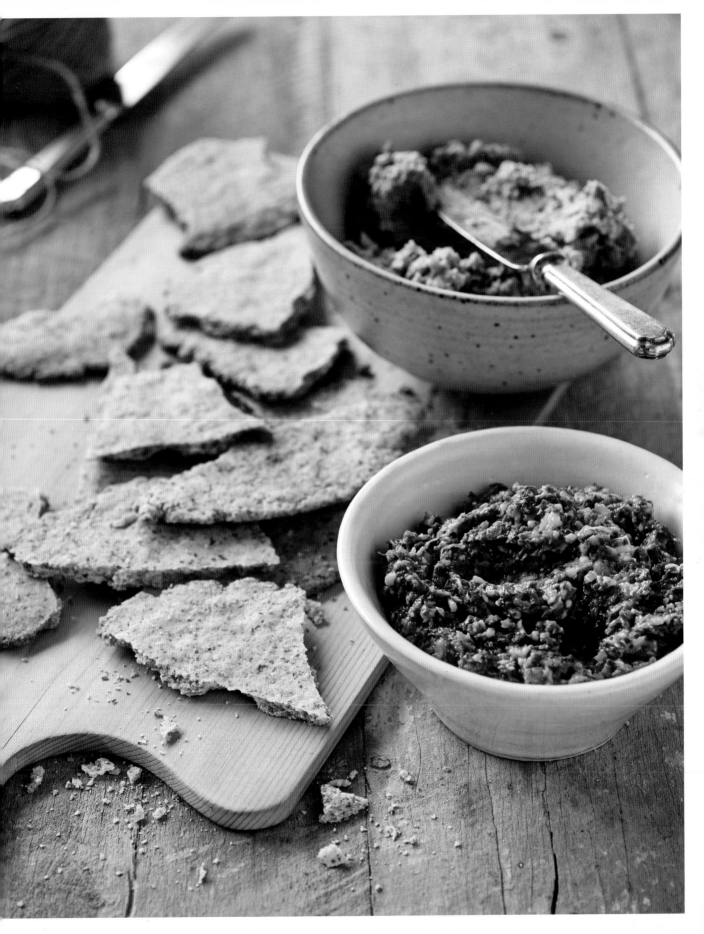

GREEK TZATZIKI

▲WF ▲GF ▲SF ▲VG   MAKES 2 CUPS

If you've been living under the Parthenon for the last few years, and are unfamiliar with this traditional Greek appetiser, it's basically cucumber with Greek-style yoghurt and a whole bunch of medicinal ingredients stirred in to make your skin glow. Opa!

1 fresh cucumber peeled, seeds removed, and grated

pinch of Celtic sea salt

520 g (1 lb 2¹/₂ oz/2 cups) plain, additive-free Greek-style yoghurt

2 garlic cloves, minced

60 ml (2 fl oz/¹/₄ cup) extra virgin olive oil

1 tablespoon freshly squeezed lemon juice

1 tablespoon finely chopped dill

1 tablespoon finely chopped mint

Place the cucumber in a sieve over a bowl and sprinkle over the salt. Let it sit for 15 minutes.

Meanwhile, place the yoghurt, garlic, olive oil and lemon juice in a separate bowl and stir well to combine. Add the cucumber and fresh herbs and season to taste.

Cover and refrigerate for 15 minutes to allow the flavours to meld.

This tzatziki will keep in an airtight container in the fridge for 5 days.

AVOCADO AND TAHINI SPREAD

▲WF ▲DF ▲GF ▲SF ▲VG   MAKES ½ CUP

For a super speedy, nutrient-packed meal, look no further than this creamy spread. Just whizz it up, and pop it onto a good bit of gluten-free toast – I like to have mine smothered on slices of Chia and Flaxseed Loaf (see page 222). I promise that those conventional dead spreads will be out the window once you feel the health benefits and experience the scrumptious living flavours.

1 avocado, peeled and stone removed

2 tablespoons tahini

1 tablespoon freshly squeezed lemon juice

¹/₂ teaspoon Celtic sea salt

1 teaspoon apple cider vinegar

freshly ground black pepper, to taste

sunflower seeds, to serve

sesame seeds, to serve

torn basil leaves, to serve

Place the avocado, tahini, lemon juice, salt, vinegar and pepper in a food processor and blend until smooth.

Serve on chia and flaxseed bread, with some sunflower and/or sesame seeds and some basil on top, for the ultimate snack.

This dip will keep for 5 days in an airtight container in the fridge.

ZUCCHINI HUMMUS

▲WF ▲DF ▲GF ▲SF ▲VG   MAKES 2–3 CUPS

A beautiful dip which is perfectly paired with crunchy flat bread. This healing combination is my food crush of the moment.

1 green zucchini (courgette), peeled and roughly chopped

160 g (5¹/₂ oz/1 cup) almonds, soaked in water for 30 minutes

60 ml (2 fl oz/¹/₄ cup) freshly squeezed lemon juice

¹/₂ teaspoon grated lemon zest

2 garlic cloves, minced

1 tablespoon ground cumin

1 teaspoon Celtic sea salt

¹/₂ teaspoon freshly ground black pepper

2 tablespoons tahini

60 ml (2 fl oz/¹/₄ cup) extra virgin olive oil

1 small handful of flat-leaf (Italian) parsley, leaves only

Put the zucchini, almonds, lemon juice and zest, garlic, cumin, salt and pepper in a food processor and process until smooth.

Add the tahini and olive oil and pulse just a few times.

Add the parsley and pulse a further couple of times.

This will keep in an airtight container in the fridge for 5 days.

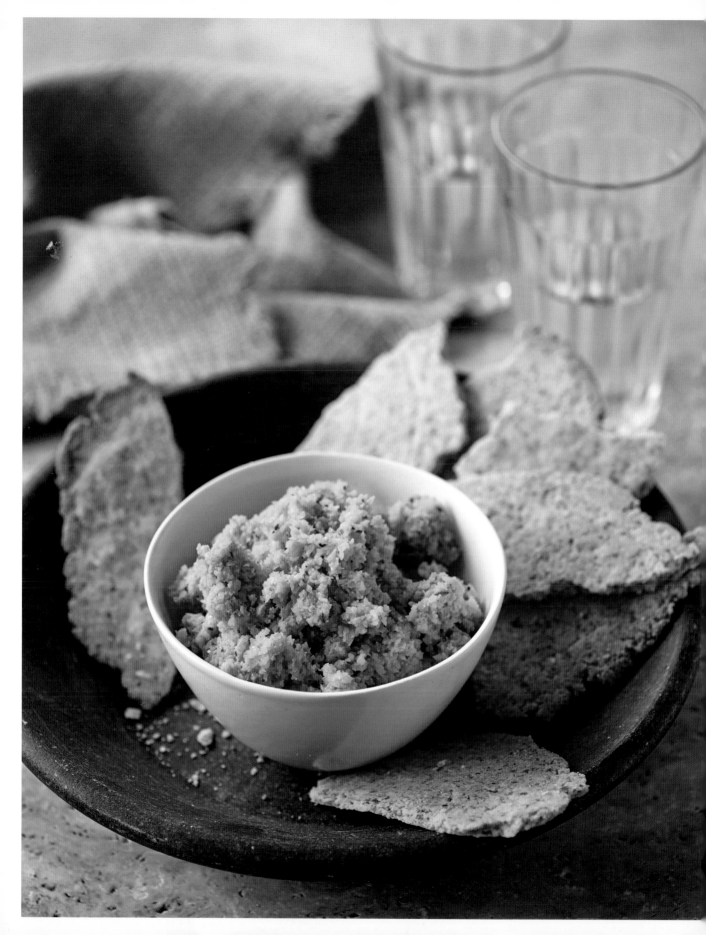

ROASTED CAULIFLOWER DIP

▲WF ▲DF ▲GF ▲SF ▲VG   MAKES 2 CUPS

White bundles of floret happiness are what make up this roasted dip. The additional spices will provide a depth of flavour and the garlic and lemon gives it zing.

1 teaspoon ground turmeric

1 teaspoon ground coriander (see note)

1 teaspoon mild paprika

1 teaspoon ground cumin

1 teaspoon dried oregano

pinch of Celtic sea salt

2 garlic cloves, minced

60 ml (2 fl oz/1/4 cup) freshly squeezed
  lemon juice

80 ml (2 1/2 fl oz/1/3 cup) extra virgin olive oil

1/2 head of a large cauliflower, cut into florets

freshly ground black pepper, to taste

Preheat the oven to 175°C (345°F/Gas 3–4).

Mix the spices, oregano, salt, garlic and lemon juice together in a bowl. Add the olive oil to make a paste. Add the cauliflower and swirl around until evenly coated. Place on a baking tray and season with black pepper.

Transfer to the oven and bake for 35–40 minutes. Remove from the oven and allow to cool.

Once cooled, transfer to a food processor and blend until creamy.

Refrigerate until you are ready to eat it.

This dip will keep for 5 days in the fridge in an airtight container.

NOTE: You can substitute a few sprigs of fresh coriander (cilantro) for the ground.

▶SUPERCHARGED TIP◀

For a creamier dip add 80 ml (2 1/2 fl oz/1/3 cup) almond milk at the end. For a cheesy dip add 1 tablespoon nutritional yeast flakes.

ZESTY SARDINE PÂTÉ

▲WF ▲GF ▲SF   MAKES ¹/₂ CUP

A wonderful creamy and full-flavoured spread makes this pâté a perfect topper for crackers or a dipper for cucumber, celery and carrot sticks. Or you can always dig in with a spoon and eat it straight up.

2 x 45 g (1¹/₂ oz) tin sardines in extra virgin olive oil

80 g (2³/₄ oz) unsalted butter, softened

2 garlic cloves, peeled

1 teaspoon freshly squeezed lemon juice

1 teaspoon grated lemon zest

2 teaspoons thyme leaves

Celtic sea salt and freshly ground white pepper, to taste

Place all the ingredients in a food processor and blend to a smooth paste.

This is ready to serve immediately but will keep in an airtight container in the fridge for 4 days.

▶HEALTH BENEFITS◀

Sardines are full of omega-3 fatty acids which have also been demonstrated to have potent anti-inflammatory effects. They are a great inclusion in the diet of people suffering with arthritis or joint pain.

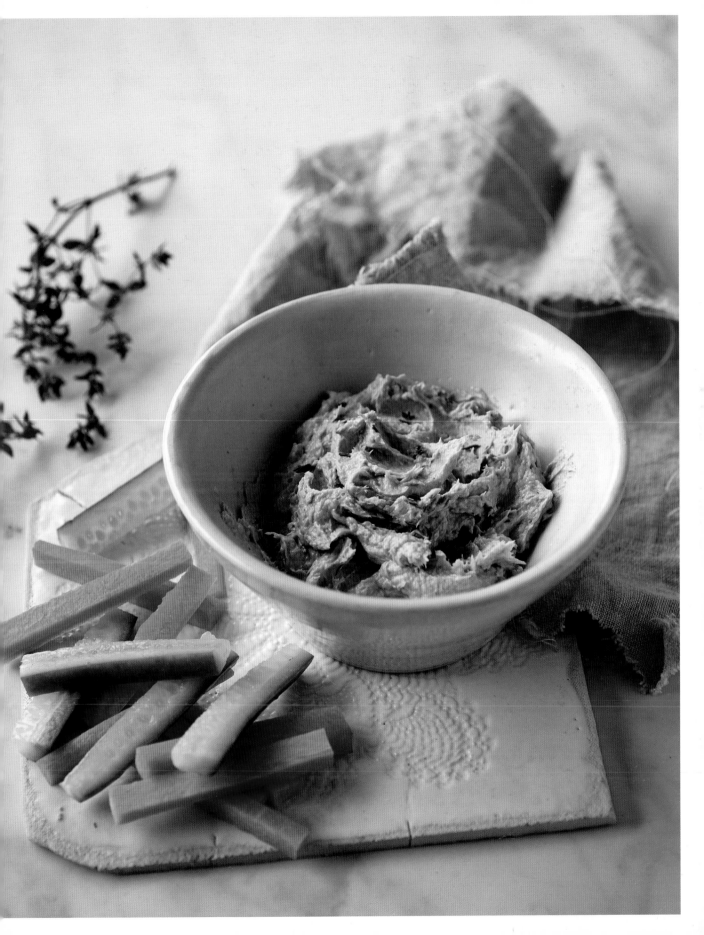

MOROCCAN HARISSA PASTE

▲WF ▲DF ▲GF ▲SF ▲VG   MAKES 1 CUP

Harissa is a hot chilli paste that is commonly found in North African cooking, mainly Moroccan, Algerian and Tunisian cuisines. It's added to couscous, soups, pastas and other recipes. It can also be purchased in Middle Eastern stores.

10 small red chillies, seeds removed

3 garlic cloves, minced

1/2 teaspoon Celtic sea salt

2 tablespoons extra virgin olive oil

1 teaspoon ground coriander

1 teaspoon ground caraway seeds

1/2 teaspoon ground cumin

Place all the ingredients in a food processor and blend until smooth.

The paste will keep in an airtight container in the fridge for up to a month. It can be reinvigorated with a dash of olive oil.

VIETNAMESE DRESSING

▲WF ▲DF ▲GF ▲SF ▲VG   MAKES 2/3 CUP

The perfect partner to an Asian dish, try this dressing over steamed Asian greens, steamed fish, healthy slaw or as a dipping sauce next to brown rice sushi. For a thicker dipping sauce add a couple of tablespoons of nut butter to the mix.

5 drops stevia liquid, or 2 tablespoons rice malt syrup or xylitol

1 small garlic clove, minced

2–3 cm (3/4–11/4 inch) piece of ginger, peeled and grated

2 tablespoons finely diced red onion

60 ml (2 fl oz/1/4 cup) filtered water

4 anchovies, finely chopped

1 tablespoon apple cider vinegar

2 tablespoons wheat-free tamari

1/2 teaspoon sesame oil

60 ml (2 fl oz/1/4 cup) freshly squeezed lime juice

Shake all the ingredients together in a jar until well combined.

The dressing will keep in an airtight jar in the fridge for 3–4 days.

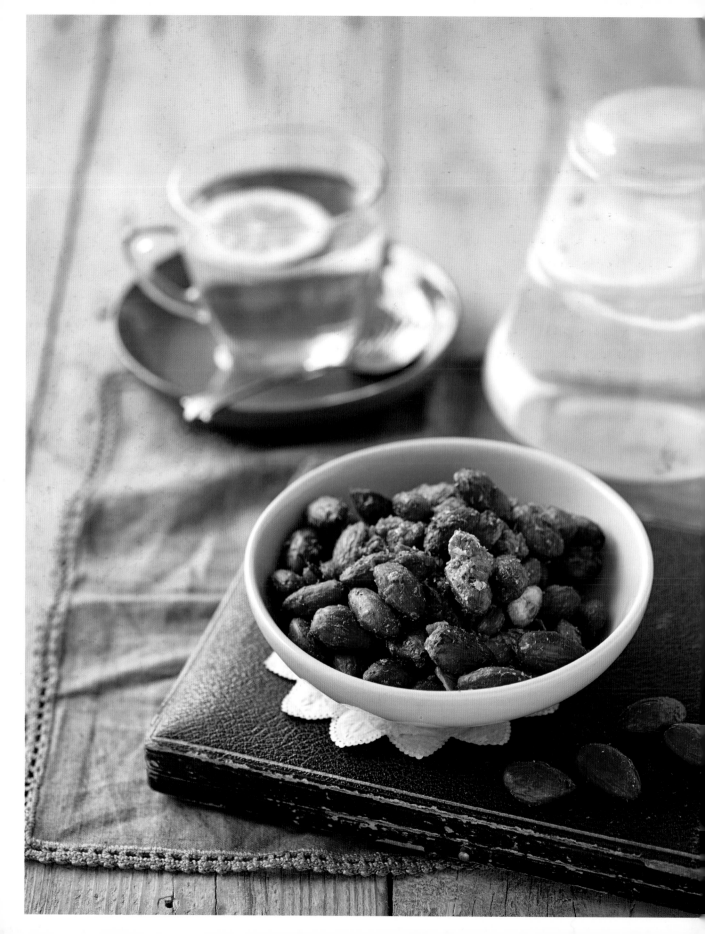

SEANUTS

▲WF ▲DF ▲GF ▲SF　　　SERVES 4

These remind me of the Asian snack ikan bilis – delicious dried anchovies often served with nuts. The addition of the sardines makes these nuts absolutely and undeniably delicious.

320 g (11¼ oz/2 cups) almonds

2 x 45 g (1½ oz) tin sardines, chopped

8 garlic cloves, sliced

2 tablespoons extra virgin olive oil

1 teaspoon Celtic sea salt

6 drops stevia liquid

2 tablespoons grated lime zest, plus extra for serving (optional)

Soak the almonds in 750 ml (26 fl oz/3 cups) filtered warm water overnight. (This step is optional.)

Preheat the oven to 200°C (400°F/Gas 6).

Place all the ingredients, except the lime zest, in a bowl and stir to combine.

Place the almond mixture on a baking tray and sprinkle with the lime zest.

Cook in the oven for 25 minutes, stirring after 15 minutes.

Remove from the oven, transfer to a bowl and serve sprinkled with additional lime zest, if desired.

The seanuts will keep for 5–7 days in an airtight container.

⬗ SUPERCHARGED TIP ⬖

If you're using tinned sardines in extra virgin olive oil you don't need to add the additional oil.

CHEESY ZUCCHINI PICCATA

▲WF ▲DF ▲GF ▲SF   SERVES 2–3

Zucchini offers your body an abundance of antioxidant-rich Vitamin C, along with iron, calcium, magnesium, phosphate and zinc. Think hair, skin and nails worthy of an Italian supermodel.

2 zucchini (courgettes), sliced into
    5 mm (1/4 inch) thick pieces

1 1/2 teaspoons Celtic sea salt

2 organic eggs, beaten

3 tablespoons nutritional yeast flakes

Preheat the oven to 200°C (400°F/Gas 6). Line a baking tray with baking paper.

Place the zucchini in a sieve over a bowl. Sprinkle the sea salt over the zucchini to draw out the moisture and let it sit for 20 minutes. (This step ensures that your chip will be crunchy.) Pat with a paper towel to thoroughly dry.

Place the eggs in a bowl. Put the yeast flakes in a separate bowl. Dip each zucchini slice in the egg and then coat it with the yeast flakes. Repeat until you have used all the zucchini slices.

Transfer to a baking tray, taking care not to crowd the tray, and cook in the oven for 20 minutes, turning after 15 minutes.

Remove from the oven and serve warm.

SALT AND VINEGAR KALE CHIPS

▲WF ▲DF ▲GF ▲SF ▲VG   SERVES 2

The addition of some spoonfuls of apple cider vinegar creates a kale chip that not only goes KAPOW in your mouth but becomes a bite packed with epic proportions of vitamins and minerals.

2 tablespoons extra virgin olive oil

1 tablespoon apple cider vinegar

1 bunch kale leaves, washed, stems
    removed, and torn into bite-sized pieces

good pinch of Celtic sea salt

Preheat the oven to 175°C (345°F/Gas 3–4).

In a large bowl, combine the olive oil and vinegar. Add the kale and ensure each piece gets coated in the oil mixture.

Transfer the kale pieces to a baking tray and cook in the oven for 15–17 minutes, turning halfway through, removing any that are already cooked.

Transfer to a bowl and enjoy warm.

TURMERIC AND ROSEMARY SWEET POTATO FRIES

▲WF ▲DF ▲GF ▲SF ▲VG   SERVES 4

I have finally mastered the art of the sweet potato fry – crispy skin on the outside meets tender orange flesh. A bowl of these will convert even the hardiest sweet-tater-hater.

2 tablespoons extra virgin olive oil

3 garlic cloves, minced

2 tablespoons ground turmeric

2 teaspoons rosemary

1 teaspoon Celtic sea salt

grind of black pepper

1 large sweet potato, washed, peeled and cut into 1 cm (½ inch) fries

Preheat the oven to 200°C (400°F/Gas 6) and line a baking tray with baking paper.

Mix the olive oil, garlic, turmeric, rosemary, salt and pepper together in a large bowl.

Add the sweet potato fries to the bowl and stir until they are evenly coated in the oil.

Place on the baking tray, ensuring they are widely spread out. Cook in the oven for 45 minutes, turning after 20 minutes.

Remove from the oven and serve warm.

▶HEALTH BENEFITS◀

Orange root vegetables such as sweet potato contain beta-carotene, which converts to Vitamin A when digested, promoting hair growth and improving the circulation of oxygen to the hair follicles.

STUFFED MUSHROOMS WITH PISTACHIOS

▲WF ▲DF ▲GF ▲SF ▲VG   SERVES 4

The perfect entrée or a light meal on their own, stuffed mushrooms will really take your taste buds to town with their delicious combination of nuttiness and flavour.

16 button mushrooms or 8 large Swiss browns, washed and stems removed

MARINADE

2 tablespoons wheat-free tamari

2 tablespoons extra virgin olive oil

2 garlic cloves, minced

1 tablespoon apple cider vinegar

20 g (3/4 oz/2/3 cup) chopped flat-leaf (Italian) parsley

STUFFING

100 g (3 1/2 oz/3/4 cup) finely chopped pistachios

freshly ground black pepper

1 tablespoon extra virgin olive oil

Place the mushrooms in a large bowl and steep them in hot water briefly. Pat dry with a paper towel. (This step will help the mushrooms soak up the marinade.)

Mix the marinade ingredients together in a bowl.

Add the mushrooms to the marinade mix, ensuring each mushroom is well coated, and leave them to marinate in the fridge for 1 hour.

Preheat the oven to 180°C (350°F/Gas 4).

Meanwhile, mix the stuffing ingredients together in a bowl.

Remove the mushrooms from the fridge and transfer to a baking tray, cap side up. Divide the stuffing mixture among the mushroom caps.

Transfer to the oven and cook for 20 minutes.

Serve immediately.

▶HEALTH BENEFITS◀

Mushrooms truly are a magic medicine food with immune-enhancing and anti-inflammatory effects.

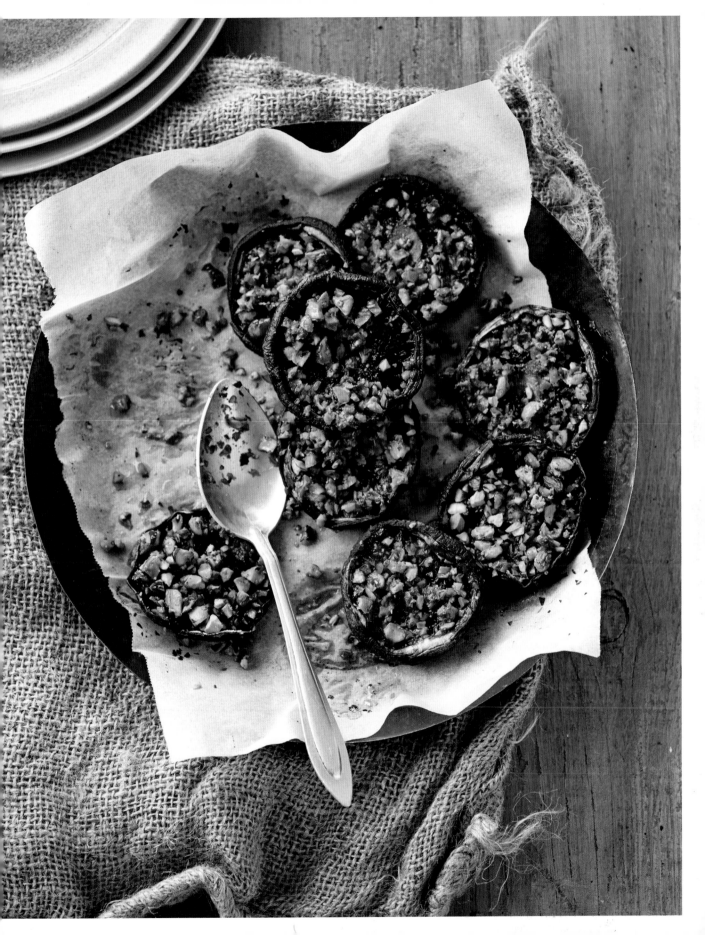

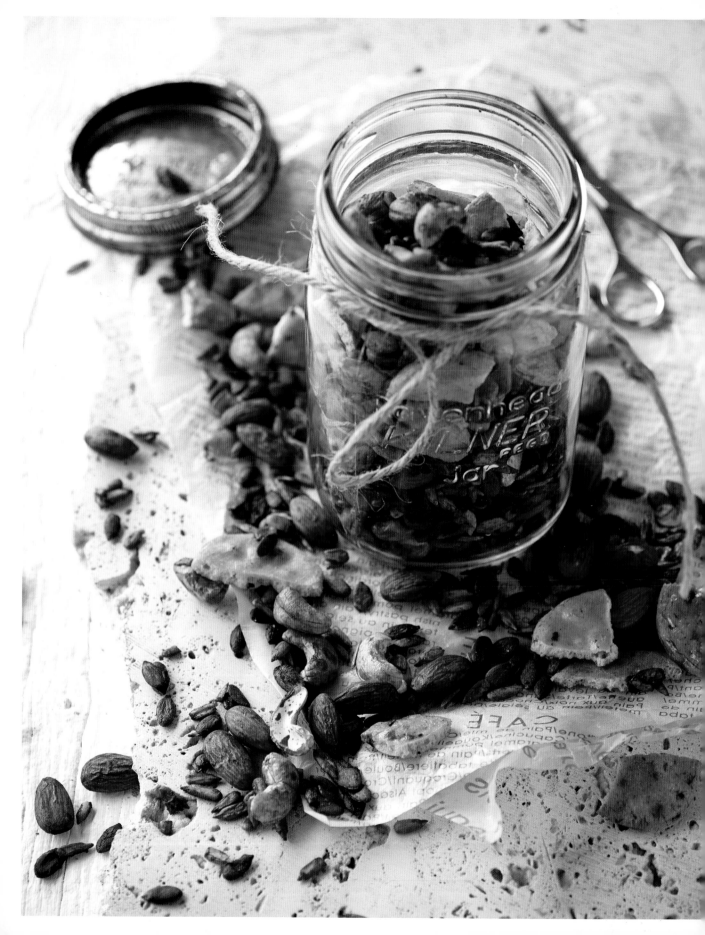

TAMARI NIBBLE MIX

▲WF ▲DF ▲GF ▲SF ▲VG   SERVES 4

Tired of reaching into your handbag and finding the same old ho-hum snack? Here's a quick-fix recipe to help you mix things up a little. It's full of good fats and B vitamins so your body and mind will love it too.

160 g (5^1/2 oz/1 cup) almonds

155 g (5^1/2 oz/1 cup) raw cashew nuts

75 g (2^1/2 oz/^{1}/2 cup) pepitas (pumpkin seeds)

75 g (2^1/2 oz/^{1}/2 cup) sunflower seeds

60 ml (2 fl oz/^{1}/4 cup) wheat-free tamari

90 g (3^1/4 oz) additive-free brown rice crackers, broken into bite-sized pieces

Preheat the oven to 160°C (315°F/Gas 2–3) and line a baking tray with baking paper.

Place the nuts and seeds in a bowl and mix to combine. Pour over the tamari, and mix so the seeds are well coated. Transfer to the baking tray and cook in the oven for 25 minutes.

Remove from the oven and cool. Add the rice crackers before serving.

Store in an airtight container for up to 2 weeks until ready to bag.

ROASTED ROOT VEGETABLES

▲WF ▲DF ▲GF ▲SF ▲VG   SERVES 4

Root vegetables like carrots, sweet potato, parsnips, turnips, garlic and onions are not only inexpensive, they are also loaded with health benefits. This magical mixture of autumn vegetables will fill you up with skin loving beta-carotene and Vitamin C.

1 butternut pumpkin (squash), peeled and chopped into 2.5 cm (1 inch) pieces

1 small sweet potato, peeled and chopped into 2.5 cm (1 inch) pieces

2 turnips, peeled and chopped into 2.5 cm (1 inch) pieces

3 carrots, peeled and chopped into 2.5 cm (1 inch) pieces

3 zucchini (courgettes), chopped into 2.5 cm (1 inch) pieces

1 brown onion, quartered

1 garlic bulb, cloves separated and peeled

large pinch of Celtic sea salt

freshly ground black pepper, to taste

60 ml (2 fl oz/¼ cup) extra virgin olive oil

chopped herbs, such as rosemary or thyme, to serve

Preheat the oven to 220°C (425°F/Gas 7).

Grease a large baking tray and add all the vegetables, except the garlic, to the tray, remembering not to crowd them. Splash over the olive oil and sprinkle with salt and pepper.

Transfer to the oven and cook for 20 minutes. Remove, turn the vegetables, and add the garlic. Return to the oven and cook for a further 35 minutes, or until the vegetables are golden brown, turning them occasionally.

Remove from the oven and sprinkle over the fresh herbs before serving.

DEHYDRATED SPICY SEEDS

▲WF ▲DF ▲GF ▲SF ▲VG   MAKES 1½ CUPS

Seeds are an excellent source of protein, as well as adding texture and flavour to your meals. Combined with the anti-inflammatory power of turmeric you can turn to these appetisers, lunchbox fillers, toppers or snacks whenever the mood takes you.

1 tomato

1 tablespoon xylitol, or ⅛ teaspoon stevia powder

1 teaspoon mild paprika

1 teaspoon ground turmeric

2 teaspoons wheat-free tamari

1 teaspoon Celtic sea salt

2 tablespoons flaxseed oil

220 g (7¾ oz/1½ cups) pumpkin and sunflower seeds (can be soaked and drained)

Preheat the oven to 45°C (113°F/Gas ¼).

Place all the ingredients, except the seeds, in a food processor and process until well combined.

Stir in the seeds, ensuring they are well coated in the sauce.

Transfer to a baking tray and dehydrate them in the oven, with the door partially open, for 8 hours, or until they are dry and crisp.

These will keep in an airtight container for 2–3 months.

NOTE: To dehydrate is to draw the moisture out of the food by way of slow cooking on a very low temperature under 50°C (122°F).

▶SUPERCHARGED TIP◀

Soak the seeds overnight if you have the time. If you own a dehydrator, place them on trays at 45°C (113°F) for 8–10 hours. Soaking and dehydrating the seeds makes them more digestible and also increases the nutritional content.

BROCCOLINI WITH GARLIC AND CHILLI

▲WF ▲DF ▲GF ▲SF ▲VG   SERVES 4

When time is of the essence and tummies are rumbling, a quick-as-a-flash green veggie dish is ideal to stoke up the embers. Pile this on your plate and your appetite will soon be satisfied.

2 bunches broccolini, trimmed

2 tablespoons extra virgin olive oil

2 garlic cloves, thinly sliced

1 long red chilli, seeds removed, finely chopped

good pinch of Celtic sea salt

1 tablespoon freshly squeezed lemon juice

Place the broccolini in a bamboo steamer over a saucepan of simmering water, and steam for 5–7 minutes, until tender.

Heat the olive oil in a frying pan over medium heat. Add the garlic and chilli and sauté for a few minutes. Add the broccolini, sprinkle with salt, and stir until warmed through. Add the lemon juice and serve hot.

▶HEALTH BENEFITS◀

Fresh broccolini is a particularly rich source of the anti-inflammatory phytonutrients, kaempferol and isothiocyanates. Research has shown that the presence of kaempferol can lessen the impact of allergy-related substances on our body. Broccolini contains significant amounts of anti-inflammatory omega-3 fatty acids, too.

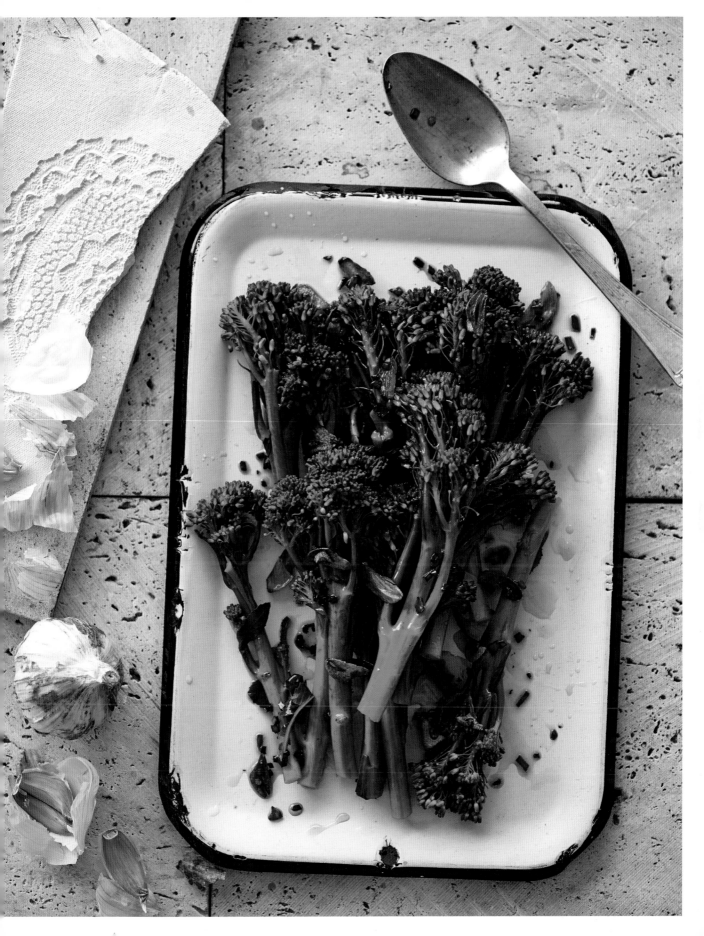

BROWN RICE SUSHI

▲WF ▲DF ▲GF ▲SF   SERVES 4

Delicious and fun to make, brown rice sushi is not as complex as one might expect. Try this extremely simple recipe with an easy-going method, healthy ingredients and light-hearted playfulness. If you're looking for a neighbouring dipping sauce, try partnering these with Vietnamese Dressing (see page 97) or some wheat-free tamari and ginger pickled in apple cider vinegar.

370 g (12¾ oz/2 cups) cooked brown rice, cooled

2 tablespoons apple cider vinegar

2 tablespoons wheat-free tamari

2 tablespoons tahini

75 g (2½ oz/½ cup) sesame seeds

1 x 25 g (1 oz) 10-sheet packet nori sheets

1 avocado, peeled, stone removed, and chopped

425 g (15 oz) tin tuna, drained

Place the cooked rice in a bowl and add the vinegar, tamari, tahini and sesame seeds.

Lay a nori sheet on top of a sushi mat and spoon the rice mixture over half the square, so the mixture is approximately 2 cm (¾ inch) thick. Using a large spoon, add some tuna and avocado, ensuring that the rice mixture is covered. Using the sushi mat, roll up the sushi as tightly as possible. Wet each end of the rolled sushi with a little water to ensure it sticks together.

Repeat this process until all the mixture has been used.

Use a sharp knife, dipped in water, to cut the sushi into 4 cm (1½ inch) segments.

Place in the fridge for 30 minutes to meld the ingredients together.

▶HEALTH BENEFITS◀

Brown rice is rich in zinc and magnesium and the perfect skin and hair hero.

SWEET POTATO HASH

▲WF ▲GF ▲SF   SERVES 4

Sweeter than standard hash browns, this dish can be made with minimal effort and will keep the family smiling.

1 large sweet potato, peeled and grated

1 small onion, thinly sliced

1 teaspoon ground cumin

pinch of Celtic sea salt

freshly ground black pepper

2 organic eggs, lightly whisked

1 tablespoon extra virgin olive oil

40 g (1½ oz/½ cup) grated parmesan cheese (see note)

Preheat the oven to 220°C (425°F/Gas 7).

In a medium bowl, combine the sweet potato, onion, cumin, salt, pepper and eggs.

Using your hands, squeeze out any excess moisture and spread the mixture over a baking tray. Sprinkle the parmesan cheese or nutritional yeast flakes over the mixture and cook in the oven for 30 minutes, or until crispy.

Remove from the oven, cut into 4 large (or 8 small) slices and serve hot.

NOTE: For a dairy-free option, substitute the cheese with 3 tablespoons nutritional yeast flakes.

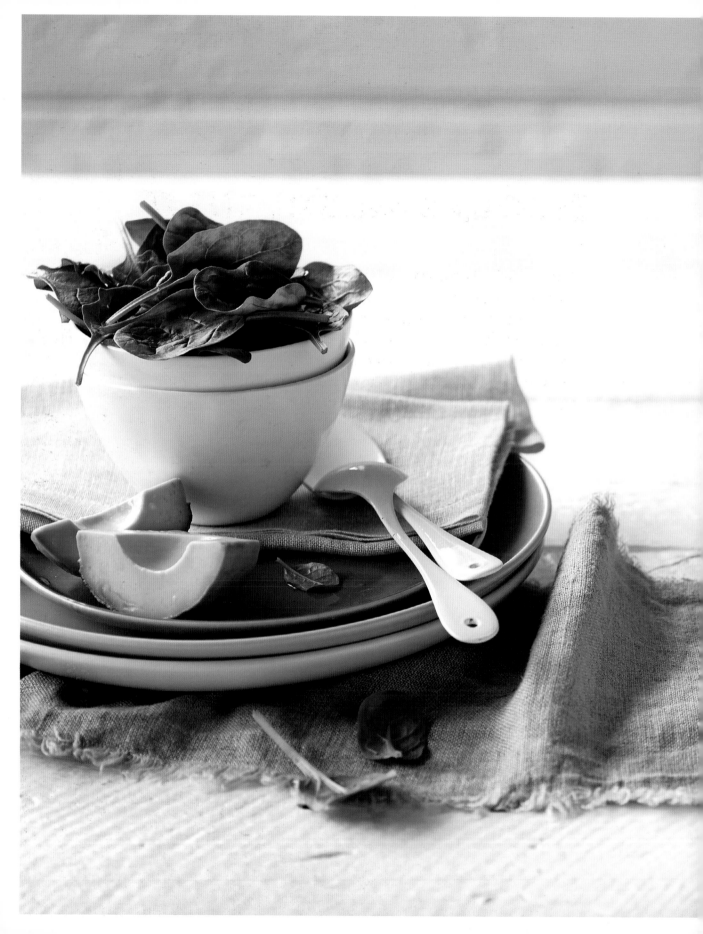

SOUPS AND SALADS

Cup-a-soup is for mugs. You'll adore this selection of health-restoring rustic soups, best served in a wide-mouthed bowl with a large rounded spoon for easy slurpability. From red and green salads and simple slaws to feisty Asian-inspired choices, make the most of salad season with these gorgeous bowls of fresh and earthy produce, guaranteed to beautify.

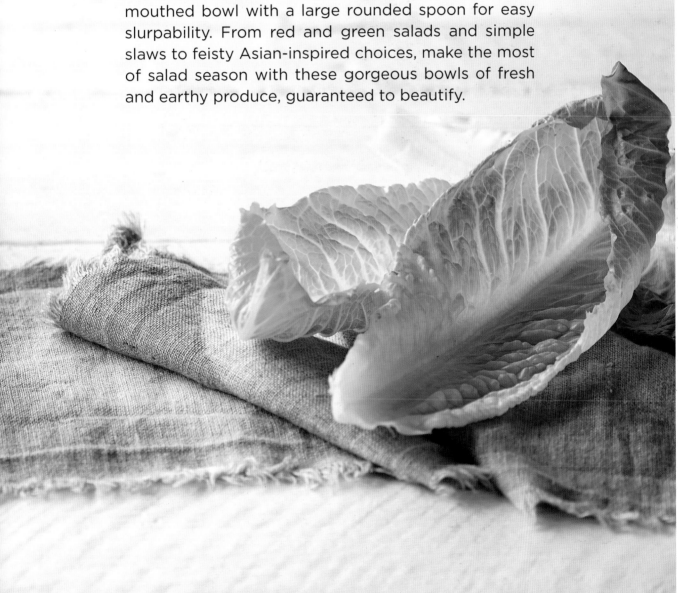

MOROCCAN LAMB SOUP

▲WF ▲DF ▲GF ▲SF   SERVES 4-5

As the weather chills, it's a good time to pluck your soup pot from its nesting place and bring the tastes of western North Africa to your home. Feast your eyes upon all the delicious flavoursome and nutritious ingredients and eat to your heart's content.

2 tablespoons extra virgin olive oil

1 kg (2 lb 4 oz) diced lamb (shoulder or leg), fat trimmed

1 brown onion, thinly sliced

1 tablespoon ground turmeric

1 tablespoon ground ginger

1 tablespoon ground cinnamon

1 tablespoon harissa

215 g (7½ oz/1 cup) lentils

2 litres (70 fl oz/8 cups) homemade chicken stock

1 organic egg (optional)

1 large tomato, diced

1 bunch baby English spinach leaves

juice of 1 lemon

1 bunch coriander (cilantro), leaves only, to serve

Heat 1 tablespoon of the olive oil in a frying pan over high heat and sear the lamb for 5 minutes. Remove from the heat and set aside.

Add the remaining oil to a large saucepan over high heat. Add the onion and cook for 3 minutes, stirring, until the onion has caramelised. Reduce the heat to medium and add the turmeric, ginger and cinnamon to the pan and cook for a few minutes. Add the lamb to the pan and stir. Add the harissa and lentils and stir well. Add the chicken stock, reduce the heat, and simmer, covered, for 1 hour or until the lamb is tender.

In a cup, lightly whisk the egg (if using). Whisk it into the soup mixture, stirring constantly. Add the tomato, lemon juice and English spinach and simmer for 5 minutes.

Serve in bowls, topped with the coriander.

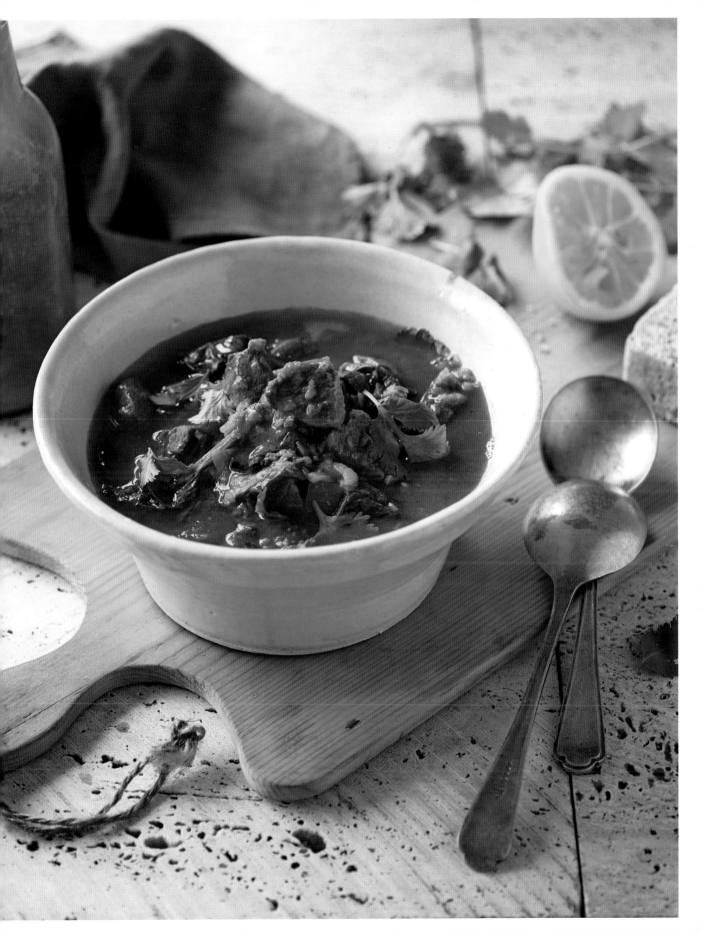

SWEET POTATO AND SPINACH SOUP

▲WF ▲DF ▲GF ▲SF   SERVES 4

Having a meatless Monday? Why not fill it up with a deliciously creamy, sweet potato, all-round family-friendly soup? It's a whole lot cheaper than tinned, boxed or frozen soup which is typically riddled with additives, artificial flavours and sodium. The addition of coconut milk gives the soup its creamy, velvety texture.

1 large sweet potato, peeled and diced

1 tablespoon extra virgin olive oil

3 garlic cloves, minced

4–5 bunches baby English spinach leaves

500 ml (17 fl oz/2 cups) homemade or additive- and yeast-free chicken or vegetable stock

125 ml (4 fl oz/$1/2$ cup) additive-free coconut milk

$1/2$ teaspoon chopped dill

$1/2$ teaspoon Celtic sea salt

freshly ground black pepper, to taste

pinch of freshly grated nutmeg

Add enough water to a large saucepan so it's three-quarters full. Bring to the boil and add the sweet potato. Cook for 15–20 minutes, or until tender. Drain and set aside.

Meanwhile, add the olive oil to a frying pan over medium heat and sauté the garlic for 3 minutes. Add the spinach and cook for about 5 minutes, or until the spinach has wilted.

Transfer the spinach and sweet potato to a food processor. Add the stock and blend until smooth.

Transfer to a large saucepan. Add the coconut milk and dill and cook over medium heat for about 5 minutes. Season with salt and pepper to taste.

Serve in a bowl with the nutmeg sprinkled on top.

NOTE: For a vegetarian option, use vegetable stock instead of chicken.

▶HEALTH BENEFITS◀

Sweet potatoes are rich in Vitamins C and E. These are potent antioxidant vitamins that play an important role in disease prevention and longevity.

CREAMY PUMPKIN SOUP

▲WF ▲DF ▲GF ▲SF ▲VG   SERVES 3

1 tablespoon coconut oil

1 onion, diced

2 garlic cloves, minced

1/2 teaspoon finely chopped ginger

620 g (1 lb 6 oz/4 cups) finely
   chopped pumpkin

375 ml (13 fl oz/1 1/2 cups) vegetable stock

500 ml (17 fl oz/2 cups) additive-free
   coconut milk

1/2 teaspoon freshly grated nutmeg

Celtic sea salt and freshly ground black
   pepper, to taste

Heat the coconut oil in a large saucepan over medium heat. Add the onion and garlic and cook for 5–7 minutes, or until the onion is translucent. Add the remaining ingredients, stir to combine and bring to the boil. Reduce the heat and simmer for 15 minutes.

Transfer to a processor and blend until smooth.

IMMUNE-BOOSTING ROASTED GARLIC SOUP

▲WF ▲GF ▲SF ▲VG   SERVES 3

Forget the flu shot and sample an injection of empowering and immune-boosting garlic soup as ammo this winter season instead. Fight off bacteria in a single dose and keep pesky colds and the flu at bay. Bursting with goodness, every spoonful of garlic is a life-extender, so make this soup a keeper in the kitchen.

3 garlic bulbs, whole, unpeeled

2 tablespoons extra virgin olive oil

40 g (1¹/₂ oz) unsalted butter

1 large brown onion, finely chopped

1 litre (35 fl oz/4 cups) homemade vegetable or chicken stock

¹/₂ teaspoon ground turmeric

¹/₂ teaspoon ground cumin

60 ml (2 fl oz/¹/₄ cup) apple cider vinegar

1 teaspoon Celtic sea salt

freshly ground black pepper

1 teaspoon dried mixed herbs, such as oregano, thyme and sage (optional)

60 ml (2 fl oz/¹/₄ cup) additive-free coconut milk (optional, see note)

Preheat the oven to 175°C (345°F/Gas 3–4).

Cut the top off each garlic bulb, place on a baking tray and drizzle with the olive oil. Transfer to the oven and cook for 45 minutes. Remove and leave to cool.

Once cooled, squeeze the garlic cloves out of their skins into a small bowl. Transfer to a food processor and whizz for a few seconds. Set aside.

Meanwhile, heat the butter in a large saucepan over medium heat. Add the onions and sauté for 10–15 minutes, or until translucent. Stir in the chicken stock, turmeric, cumin, vinegar, blended garlic, salt, pepper and herbs, if using, and bring to the boil. Reduce the heat to medium–low, cover and cook for 30 minutes. Serve hot.

NOTE: If you would like a creamier soup, stir in the coconut milk just before serving, and heat through.

▶ **SUPERCHARGED TIP** ◀

Roasting the garlic first will provide a mellow, sweet flavour so you can sip and slurp with wild abandon.

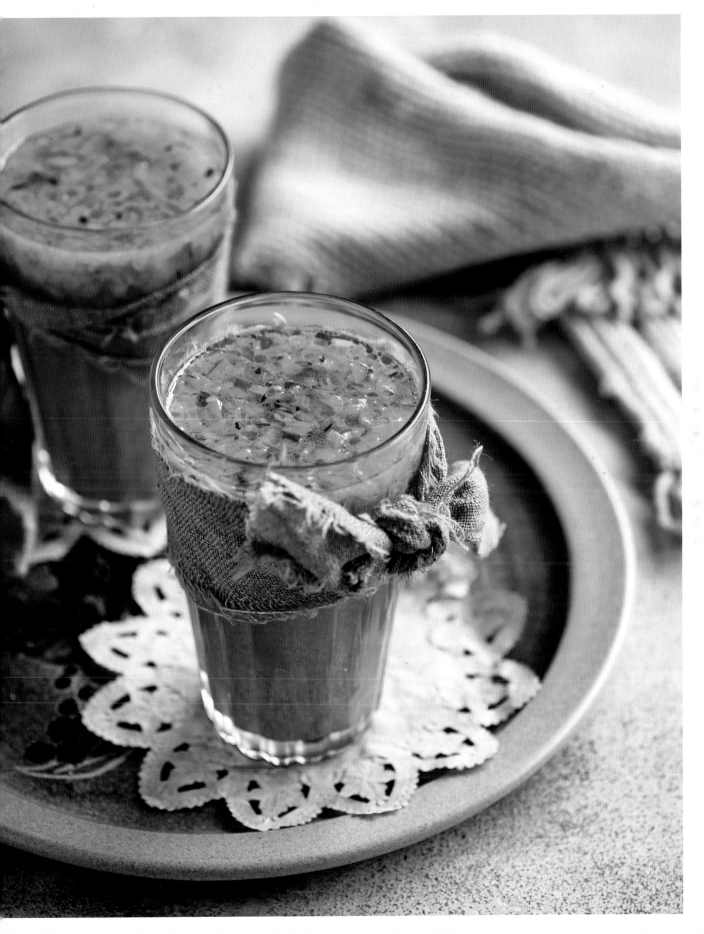

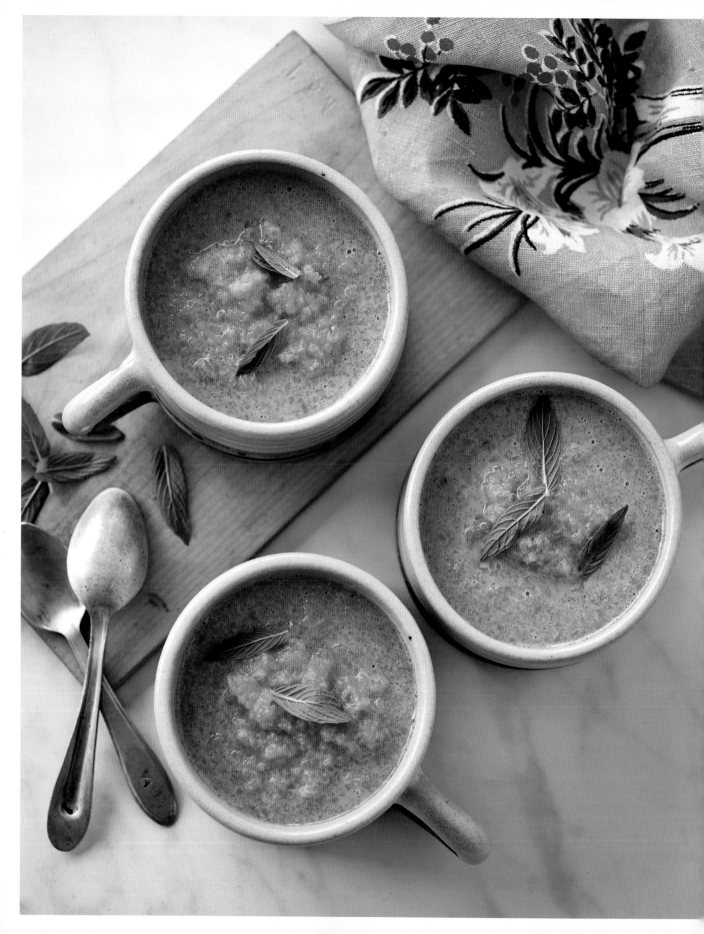

CARROT, LEMON AND FRESH MINT SOUP

▲WF ▲DF ▲GF ▲SF ▲VG   SERVES 5

Ring in the cooler weather with a carrot, lemon and mint soup with stomach-soothing ginger.
For a healthy, glowing age-proof skin indulge in this Vitamin C- and antioxidant-rich soup weekly.

12 carrots, chopped into chunks

270 ml (9¹/2 fl oz) additive-free coconut milk

1 litre (35 fl oz/4 cups) homemade vegetable stock

1 tablespoon extra virgin olive oil

1 brown onion, chopped

3 garlic cloves, minced

2.5 cm (1 inch) piece of ginger, peeled and grated

1 tablespoon Celtic sea salt

¹/2 teaspoon ground cumin

¹/2 teaspoon ground cinnamon

80 ml (2¹/2 fl oz/¹/3 cup) freshly squeezed lemon juice

2 tablespoons fresh mint, to serve

Add the carrots to a saucepan of boiling water and cook for 10–15 minutes, or until tender. Drain.

Place in a food processor with the coconut milk and stock and blend until creamy.

Meanwhile, heat a large saucepan over medium heat. Add the olive oil and sauté the onion and garlic for 5–7 minutes, or until translucent. Add the ginger and cook for a further minute, then add the salt, cumin, cinnamon, lemon juice and carrot mixture. Stir until warmed through.

Serve in bowls, topped with the mint.

SUPERFOOD SOUP

▲WF ▲DF ▲GF ▲SF ▲VG   SERVES 3-4

For an all-access backstage pass to beauty here's a superfood soup that really fits the bill.

1 tablespoon coconut oil

1 onion, diced

2 garlic cloves, minced

1/2 teaspoon finely chopped ginger

1 bunch kale leaves, washed and
   stems removed

60 g (2¼ oz/1 cup) roughly
   chopped broccoli

1 bunch English spinach leaves

1 bunch bok choy (pak choy)

155 g (5½ oz/1 cup) diced butternut
   pumpkin (squash)

1 litre (35 fl oz/4 cups) homemade
   vegetable stock

250 ml (9 fl oz/1 cup) additive-free
   coconut milk

1 tablespoon nutritional yeast flakes

Heat the coconut oil in a large saucepan over medium heat. Add the onion and garlic and cook for 5–7 minutes, or until the onion is translucent. Add the ginger and green vegetables and sweat for 3–4 minutes. Add the pumpkin and stock and bring to the boil. Reduce the heat to low, add the coconut milk and cook for a further 20 minutes.

Transfer to a food processor and blend until smooth. Serve sprinkled with nutritional yeast flakes.

▶SUPERCHARGED TIP◀

When looking for kale, seek out bunches with firm, shiny leaves and moist, snappy stems.

CHICKEN SOUP WITH LENTILS AND TURMERIC

▲WF ▲DF ▲GF ▲SF   SERVES 4

A little dash of cayenne kicks this hearty soup up a notch. It's the perfect make-ahead recipe if you want to enjoy it to wind down on a weeknight. Chicken provides an essential protein for hair strength and scalp health.

60 ml (2 fl oz/¼ cup) extra virgin olive oil

1 small onion, diced

2.5 cm (1 inch) piece of ginger, peeled and grated

3 garlic cloves, minced

1 teaspoon ground cumin

1 teaspoon ground turmeric

pinch of cayenne pepper

freshly ground black pepper

2 celery stalks, diced

3 carrots, diced

2 turnips, diced into 2.5 cm (1 inch) pieces

170 g (5¾ oz/¾ cup) lentils, rinsed or 400 g (14 oz) tin lentils

1.25 litres (44 fl oz/5 cups) homemade chicken stock

2 tablespoons apple cider vinegar

2 skinless chicken breast fillets, cut into thin strips

coriander (cilantro) leaves, to serve

Add the olive oil to a heavy-based saucepan over medium heat. Add the onion and ginger and sauté for 5–7 minutes, or until soft. Add the garlic, cumin, turmeric, cayenne pepper and black pepper and cook for a further 1 minute. Add the celery, carrots, turnips, lentils, stock and vinegar and bring to the boil. Reduce the heat and simmer, covered, for 35 minutes, or until the lentils are nearly ready. Season.

Add the chicken to the soup and cook for a further 10 minutes, or until the chicken has cooked through.

Serve hot, topped with the coriander leaves.

▶ HEALTH BENEFITS ◀

Lentils offer a valuable amount of iron, along with plenty of folate and protein. They're also a very good source of niacin and potassium.

SPINACH AND CELERY SOUP

▲WF ▲DF ▲GF ▲SF   SERVES 4

Master chef Louis P. De Gouy summed it up in 1949: 'There is nothing like a plate or a bowl of hot soup, its wisp of aromatic steam making the nostrils quiver with anticipation, to dispel the depressing effects of a gruelling day at the office or the shop, rain or snow in the streets, or bad news in the papers.'

1 tablespoon extra virgin olive oil

1 large brown onion, chopped

3 garlic cloves, finely chopped

1 bunch celery, chopped, leaves reserved, to garnish

1 tablespoon thyme leaves

1 litre (35 fl oz/4 cups) homemade chicken or vegetable stock

2 turnips, cubed

1 large bunch English spinach leaves, chopped

250 ml (9 fl oz/1 cup) additive-free coconut milk

Celtic sea salt and freshly ground black pepper

Add the olive oil to a heavy-based saucepan over medium heat. Add the onion, garlic, celery and thyme and cook, stirring occasionally, for 15 minutes, or until the celery has softened. Add the stock, turnips and spinach, increase the heat and bring to the boil. Reduce the heat and simmer uncovered for 10 minutes, or until the turnips are tender. Remove from the heat and cool.

Once cooled, ladle the mixture, in batches, into a food processor and blend until well combined. Return the soup to the saucepan, add the coconut milk and simmer for 5 minutes.

Ladle into earthenware bowls (if you have them!), garnish with celery leaves and season with salt and pepper, to taste.

NOTE: Try serving this soup with the Salt and Vinegar Kale Chips (see page 100). For a vegetarian option, use veggie stock.

CREAMY LEEK AND PARSLEY SOUP

▲WF ▲GF ▲SF ▲VG   SERVES 4

A gentle yet sassy soup due to the sweetness of the parsnips. I recommend that you partake in this simple and satisfying aromatic and warming soup on frosty, chilly nights.

40 g (1¹/₂ oz) unsalted butter

3 leeks, white part only, trimmed, washed and sliced into 5 mm (¹/₄ inch) rounds

8 parsnips, chopped

2 tablespoons olive oil

1 teaspoon Celtic sea salt

1 litre (35 fl oz/4 cups) homemade vegetable stock

1 tablespoon freshly squeezed lemon juice

1 tablespoon grated lemon zest

1 tablespoon apple cider vinegar

250 ml (9 fl oz/1 cup) additive-free coconut milk

2 large handfuls of flat-leaf (Italian) parsley, chopped (reserve a little for garnish)

Add the butter to a heavy-based saucepan over medium heat. Add the leeks and toss so they are well coated in the butter, then cook for 5–7 minutes, or until softened. Add the parsnips, olive oil and salt and stir well. Add the stock, lemon juice and zest and vinegar and bring to the boil. Add the coconut milk, reduce the heat to low, cover with a lid and simmer for 20 minutes, or until the parsnips are tender. Add the parsley, transfer to a food processor and blend until smooth.

▶HEALTH BENEFITS◀

Although not as well known as their famous counterparts, onions and garlic, leeks are significant vegetables for fighting against chronic low-level inflammatory states such as diabetes, obesity and rheumatoid arthritis. Leeks can decrease the risk for these conditions by virtue of their polyphenol and kaempferol contents.

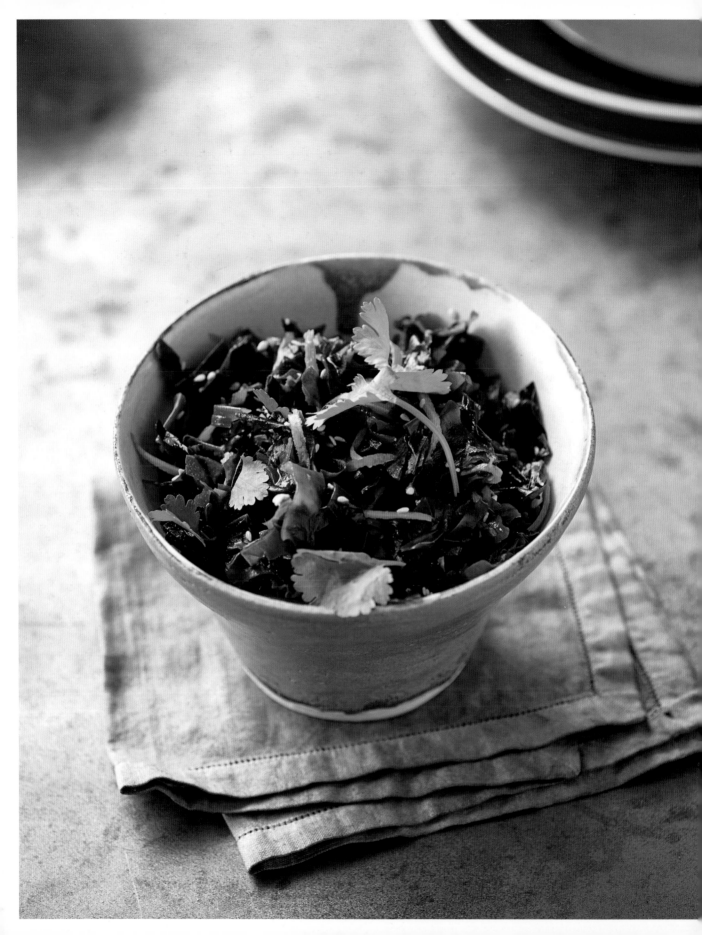

SEAWEED AND SESAME

▲WF ▲DF ▲GF ▲SF ▲VG   SERVES 4

I can't say enough good things about seaweed, but if I were to pick just one virtue it would be the ability to promote physical and mental youthfulness. Best served chilled, this healthy Japanese dish makes the perfect sidekick to fish.

25 g (1 oz) dried wakame seaweed (see note)

60 ml (2 fl oz/¼ cup) apple cider vinegar

60 ml (2 fl oz/¼ cup) wheat-free tamari

1 tablespoon sesame oil

6 drops stevia liquid

1 teaspoon freshly grated ginger

1 tablespoon freshly squeezed lemon

1 garlic clove, minced

1 carrot, grated

2 tablespoons chopped coriander (cilantro) leaves

1 tablespoon toasted sesame seeds, to serve

Place the seaweed in a small bowl and cover with water. Soak for 5 minutes, then drain and rinse under running water, squeezing out any excess water.

In a medium bowl, mix all the ingredients together, except the sesame seeds, and toss to combine well.

Sprinkle with the sesame seeds and serve.

NOTE: You can purchase seaweed at your local health food store or Asian grocer. If you are new to seaweed, you might like to start by halving the amount of seaweed in the recipe until you have worked your way into the taste.

❱HEALTH BENEFITS❰

Sea vegetables help alkalise the body and wakame seaweed is an excellent source of Vitamins A, B1, B2, B3, B5, C, E and K, folate and soluble/insoluble fibre. Seaweed has a high content of the anti-inflammatory omega-3 essential fatty acid EPA.

RED CABBAGE AND APPLE SLAW WITH TAHINI DRESSING

▲WF ▲DF ▲GF ▲VG   SERVES 2–3

1/4 red cabbage, finely shredded

1 large granny smith apple, grated

2 tablespoons chia or hemp seeds

2 celery stalks, thinly sliced

DRESSING

65 g (2$^{1}/_{4}$ oz/$^{1}/_{4}$ cup) tahini

60 ml (2 fl oz/$^{1}/_{4}$ cup) filtered water

6 drops stevia liquid

$^{1}/_{2}$ teaspoon sesame oil

good pinch of Celtic sea salt, to taste

1 tablespoon apple cider vinegar

1 tablespoon freshly squeezed lemon

In a large bowl, whisk the dressing ingredients together.

Add the salad ingredients to the bowl, toss well so they are well coated in the dressing and well combined. Serve immediately.

KALE, CARROT AND PINE NUT

▲WF ▲DF ▲GF ▲SF ▲VG   SERVES 3–4

Kale, carrot and pine nut are a scarily good combination. Use this salad as a side dish to accompany a main. I love this served alongside Keen-wah Burgers (see page 160).

1 bunch kale leaves, washed, stems
   removed, and chopped

6 carrots, grated

40 g (1 1/2 oz/1/4 cup) pine nuts

1 avocado, peeled and stone removed

1/2 red onion, thinly sliced

2 tablespoons toasted sesame seeds

DRESSING

60 ml (2 fl oz/1/4 cup) extra virgin olive oil

1 garlic clove, minced

2 tablespoons freshly squeezed lemon juice

2 teaspoons wheat-free tamari

6 drops stevia liquid (optional)

Place all the dressing ingredients in a large bowl and whisk to combine.

Put the salad ingredients in a bowl, add the dressing and serve immediately.

▶HEALTH BENEFITS◀

Kale, a cruciferous vegetable native to the Mediterranean, was one of the earliest vegetables cultivated by the ancient Egyptians and Romans. Kale contains the highest quantities of the antioxidants beta-carotene, lutein and zeaxanthin, which act as natural sun blocks from the inside out.

LAMB AND SPICED PUMPKIN SALAD

▲WF ▲GF ▲SF   SERVES 2

This is my good friend and fellow author Meredith Gaston's favourite salad. Warm salads are colourful, packed with nutrients and wonderful for digestion. The slow-roasted baby tomatoes and spiced pumpkin can be prepared in advance and warmed prior to serving to allow for quick assembly. For a dairy-free option, omit the goat's cheese.

150 g (5 1/2 oz/1 cup) cherry tomatoes

1 butternut pumpkin (squash), skin on and cut into small wedges

1/2 teaspoon ground cumin

1/2 teaspoon ground coriander

1/4 teaspoon ground cinnamon

1 tablespoon freshly grated ginger

1 tablespoon coconut oil, melted, plus extra for pan-frying

Celtic sea salt and freshly ground black pepper

3 large handfuls of mixed baby mesclun

250 g (9 oz) lamb backstrap

1 handful of basil leaves

60 g (2 1/4 oz/1/2 cup) goat's cheese

DRESSING

2 tablespoons tahini

juice of 1/2 lemon

good pinch of Celtic sea salt and freshly ground black pepper

Preheat the oven to 150°C (300°F/Gas 2).

To make the dressing, combine all the ingredients in a jug. Whisk thoroughly, gradually adding a little warm water until the dressing is smooth, thick and creamy.

Place the tomatoes on a baking tray and cook for 2–3 hours, turning every hour or so, until they are shrivelled and bursting with sweetness. This step is best done ahead of time to allow for a very quick assembly. Reheat the tomatoes slightly before serving.

Increase the oven temperature to 200°C (400°F/Gas 6). Place the pumpkin, cumin, coriander, cinnamon and ginger in a bowl and use your hands to mix well. Place the pumpkin on a baking tray, drizzle with the melted coconut oil, and season with salt and pepper. Cook in the oven for 30 minutes, or until golden and crispy.

Season the lamb. Add the coconut oil to a frying pan over medium heat and pan-fry the lamb for 3 minutes on each side (it should still be pink in the centre). Let it rest for a few minutes before slicing into 5 mm (1/4 inch) pieces.

To assemble the salad, make a bed of salad leaves and top with the warm pumpkin, lamb and tomatoes. Drizzle the tahini dressing generously over the top, scatter with the basil leaves and goat's cheese and serve warm.

▶**SUPERCHARGED TIP**◀

Lamb backstrap is a tender, grade-A cut of lamb that can be prepared simply and easily. Try pan-frying, searing, grilling (broiling), or oven roasting.

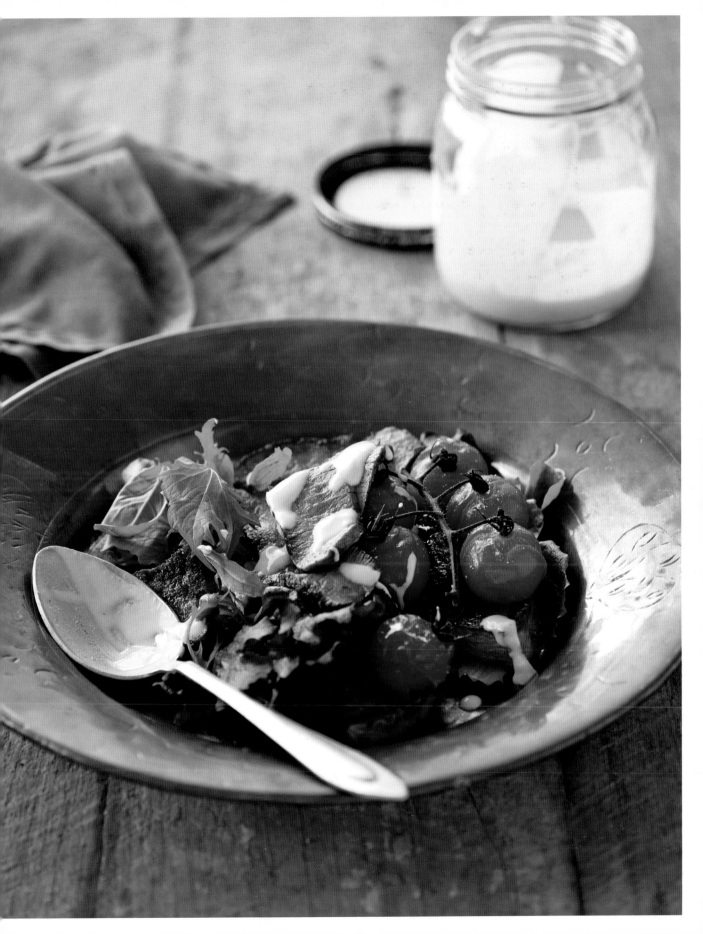

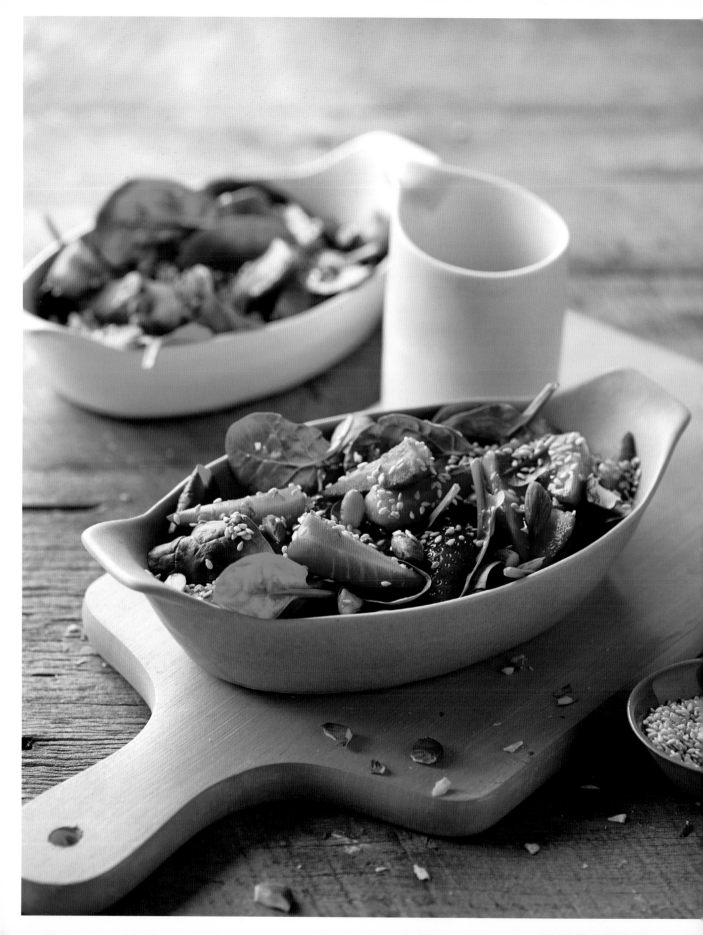

SPINACH, ALMOND AND STRAWBERRY SALAD

▲WF ▲DF ▲GF ▲VG   SERVES 2

Fresh and juicy, bursting into spring and summer months, strawberries make a surprisingly delicious addition to salads. The secret ingredient in this salad is paprika, which is sky-high in Vitamin C and antioxidants – it also contains anti-inflammatory and antibacterial properties.

1 large bunch English spinach leaves

250 g (9 oz/1²/3 cup) strawberries, hulled and quartered

80 g (2³/4 oz/¹/2 cup) almonds, toasted and coarsely chopped

2 tablespoons toasted sesame seeds

DRESSING

60 ml (2 fl oz/¹/4 cup) extra virgin olive oil

1 tablespoon apple cider vinegar

¹/4 teaspoon paprika

In a large bowl, toss the spinach, strawberries and almonds together.

In a small bowl, whisk the dressing ingredients together.

Pour the dressing over the salad, top with the sesame seeds, and serve.

CHEESY ZUCCHINI AND ASPARAGUS SALAD

▲WF ▲DF ▲GF ▲SF ▲VG   SERVES 2

An age-defying salad for all seasons. The Vitamin C content will result in a boost of your skin cells and keep collagen on side. Asparagus contains high levels of skin-clearing zinc and potassium, assisting the removal of excess fluids from the body. It has also been used to treat inflammatory conditions such as arthritis and rheumatism.

2 zucchini (courgettes)

1 bunch asparagus, trimmed

2 tablespoons nutritional yeast flakes

DRESSING

60 ml (2 fl oz/¼ cup) extra virgin olive oil

2 tablespoons freshly squeezed lemon juice

½ teaspoon Celtic sea salt

¼ teaspoon freshly ground black pepper

Preheat the oven grill (broiler) to medium.

Using a spiraliser or vegetable peeler, cut the zucchini into ribbons.

Thinly slice the asparagus on the diagonal and place under the grill (broiler) for a couple of minutes.

To make the dressing, whisk the olive oil, lemon juice, salt and pepper together in a small bowl.

Place the zucchini and asparagus in a salad bowl. Drizzle over the dressing, ensuring the vegetables are evenly coated, then sprinkle with the yeast flakes. Serve immediately.

MANGO, MACADAMIA AND ROCKET

▲WF ▲DF ▲GF ▲SF ▲VG   SERVES 4

1 bunch rocket (arugula)

1 large handful of baby English spinach
  leaves

65 g (2¼ oz) snow peas (mangetout),
  sliced on the diagonal

1 mango, peeled, stone removed, and
  chopped into cubes

1 avocado, peeled, stone removed and
  chopped into cubes

90 g (3¼ oz/⅔ cup) finely chopped
  macadamias

DRESSING

1 tablespoon freshly squeezed lime juice

grated zest of 1 lime

60 ml (2 fl oz/¼ cup) extra virgin olive oil

1 tablespoon apple cider vinegar

1 garlic clove, minced

Place the rocket, spinach and snow peas in a salad bowl.
Add the mango, avocado and macadamias and mix gently
to combine.

To make the dressing, put all the ingredients in a jar and
shake well to combine. Pour over the salad and serve.

TURMERIC, CAULIFLOWER AND ALMOND

▲WF ▲DF ▲GF ▲SF ▲VG   SERVES 4

Turmeric is a lively root, with a heady, earthy fragrance, known for its healing powers, and it can transform unglamorous, frumpy vegetables into golden anti-inflammatory bundles of wellness.

1 head of cauliflower, cut into florets

2 tablespoons extra virgin olive oil

15 g (1/2 oz/1/2 cup) chopped flat-leaf (Italian) parsley

1/2 red onion, finely diced

50 g (1 3/4 oz/1/3 cup) chopped almonds

DRESSING

80 ml (2 1/2 fl oz/1/3 cup) extra virgin olive oil

60 ml (2 fl oz/1/4 cup) freshly squeezed lemon juice

1 teaspoon grated lemon zest

1 teaspoon ground turmeric

1/2 teaspoon finely chopped ginger

1/2 teaspoon paprika

1/4 teaspoon ground cumin

1/4 teaspoon ground coriander

good pinch of Celtic sea salt

Preheat the oven to 230°C (450°F/Gas 8).

Place the cauliflower on a baking tray. Pour over the olive oil, ensuring the cauliflower is evenly coated. Cook in the oven for 30 minutes.

Place all the dressing ingredients in a jar and shake to combine.

Remove the cauliflower from the oven and place in a serving bowl. Add the parsley and onion, pour over the dressing and stir to combine well.

Serve topped with the chopped almonds.

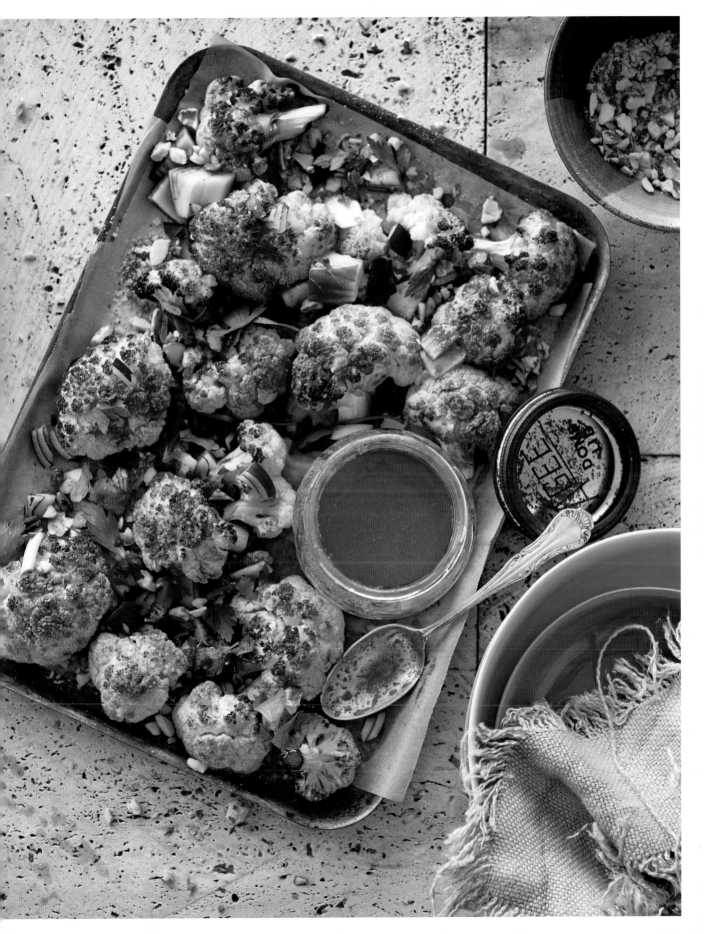

SMOKED SALMON AND BUCKWHEAT NOODLES

▲WF ▲DF ▲GF ▲SF   SERVES 2–3

1 bunch asparagus, trimmed
   and sliced on the diagonal

1 handful of snow peas (mangetout),
   chopped

250 g (9 oz) buckwheat noodles, cooked
   according to the packet instructions

1 bunch English spinach, leaves chopped

3 spring onions (scallions), thinly sliced

200 g (7 oz) smoked salmon, roughly
   chopped

1 tablespoon chia seeds

DRESSING

2 tablespoons chia oil

1¹/₂ tablespoons apple cider vinegar

1 teaspoon sesame oil

1 teaspoon wheat-free tamari

1 teaspoon freshly squeezed lemon juice

Place the asparagus and snow peas in a steamer over a saucepan of gently simmering water. Lightly steam for 7–10 minutes and then remove from the steamer to cool. Set aside.

Place all the dressing ingredients in a jar and shake well to combine.

Place the noodles, spinach, asparagus, snow peas and spring onions in a bowl and mix gently. Pour over the dressing.

Divide among the serving plates, top with the salmon and chia seeds and serve.

▶**HEALTH BENEFITS**◀

Buckwheat helps lower blood pressure and cholesterol due to its rich supply of rutin, an antioxidant phytonutrient.

ROAST PUMPKIN, BROWN RICE AND TAMARI

▲WF ▲DF ▲GF ▲SF ▲VG   SERVES 2

This colourful salad really showcases the potential of the pretty pumpkin, and even includes the seeds, which are a wonderful source of minerals. Not only will you love the sweetness of the pumpkin, you'll absolutely adore the lip-smacking dressing made with zingy lemon and apple cider vinegar, with a mildly salty tamari kick. Multiply the ingredients for the amount of mouths you need to feed and you will have a bunch of very happy and healthy campers!

600 g (1 lb 5 oz) butternut pumpkin (squash), peeled, seeds removed, cut into 2–3 cm (3/4–1 1/4 inch) pieces

extra virgin olive oil, to coat

150 g (5 1/2 oz/3/4 cup) brown long-grain rice

55 g (2 oz/1/3 cup) pepitas (pumpkin seeds)

55 g (2 oz/1/3 cup) sunflower seeds

1 1/2 tablespoons wheat-free tamari, plus 1 tablespoon extra

45 g (1 1/2 oz/1 cup) baby rocket (arugula), washed

1/2 bunch coriander (cilantro), leaves chopped, to serve

DRESSING

60 ml (2 fl oz/1/4 cup) freshly squeezed lemon juice

1 tablespoon apple cider vinegar

1 teaspoon sesame oil

1 garlic clove, minced

6 drops stevia liquid

Celtic sea salt and freshly ground black pepper, to serve

Preheat the oven to 220°C (425°F/Gas 7).

Place the pumpkin on a baking tray, coat well with olive oil and bake for about 30 minutes, turning after 15 minutes.

Meanwhile, fill a large saucepan to three-quarters full. Place over high heat and bring to the boil. Add the rice and cook for 20 minutes or until tender, but not too well cooked. Drain the rice in a sieve, rinse with cold water and set aside for 30 minutes to cool.

Place the seeds in a small bowl, drizzle with the 1 1/2 tablespoons of tamari and stir to evenly coat. Cook in a frying pan over medium–high heat for 5–10 minutes, or until lightly toasted. Remove and set aside to cool.

To make the dressing, combine the lemon juice, the 1 tablespoon of tamari, the vinegar, sesame oil, garlic, stevia and sea salt and pepper in a small jug. Whisk to combine.

Place the rice in a salad bowl. Drizzle over the dressing then add the rocket, pumpkin and tamari-coated seeds. Stir gently and serve topped with the coriander.

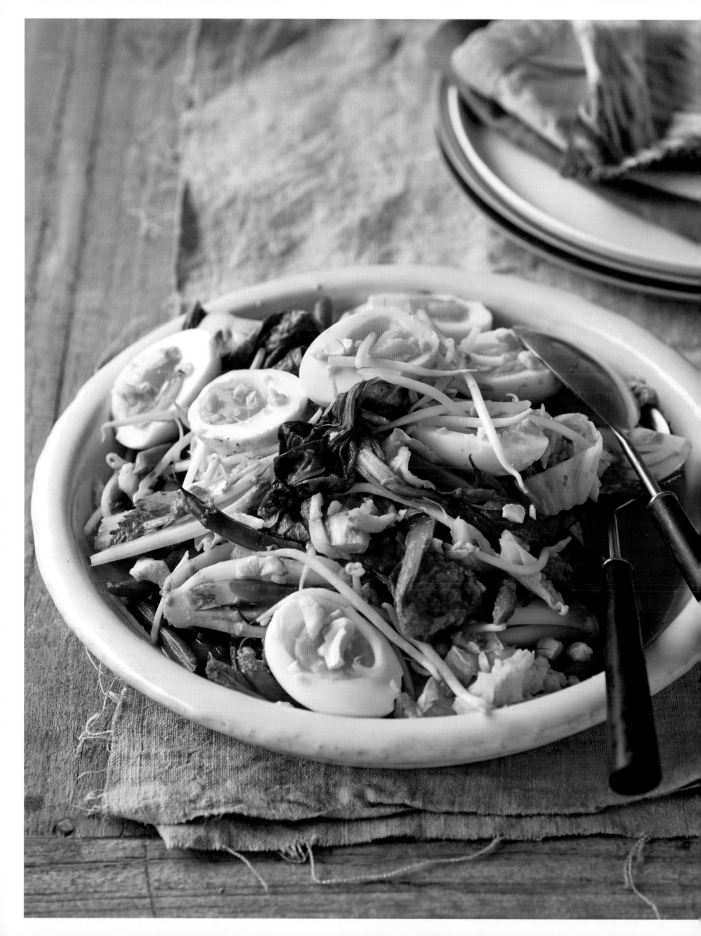

CRUNCHY GADO GADO

▲WF ▲DF ▲GF ▲SF   SERVES 2

Here's a salad that you can serve as a starter, main or even tumble into a lunchbox for work. It can be served warm or chilled. This recipe can be adapted using any vegetables you like. Some people serve it with tempeh or tofu and also topped with crushed peanuts or crunchy garlic. Just have fun with it. There are no strict rules with Gado Gado.

1/2 head of Chinese cabbage (wong bok), shredded

1 bunch bok choy (pak choy), roughly chopped

250 g (9 oz) green or snake beans, cut into 4 cm (1 1/2 inch) lengths

115 g (4 oz/1 cup) bean sprouts

4 organic boiled eggs, peeled and halved

crisp-fried garlic, to serve (optional)

1 handful of chopped nuts, such as almonds, peanuts or raw cashew nuts, to serve (optional)

GADO GADO DRESSING

1 small garlic clove, minced

2–3 cm (3/4-1 1/4 inch) piece of ginger, peeled and grated

2 tablespoons apple cider vinegar

2 tablespoons additive-free coconut milk

3 tablespoons almond or peanut butter

2 tablespoons wheat-free tamari

1/2 teaspoon sesame oil

2 tablespoons freshly squeezed lemon juice

5 drops stevia liquid

Celtic sea salt and freshly ground black pepper

Steam the vegetables over a saucepan of simmering water for 6 minutes or until they are tender.

Meanwhile, to make the dressing, place all the ingredients in a bowl and whisk until well combined. Season with salt and freshly ground black pepper.

Transfer the vegetables to a serving bowl and coat with the dressing, tossing well to combine. Top with the sprouts and eggs, sprinkle over the crispy garlic and chopped nuts, if using, and serve.

CHICKEN AND HOMEMADE MAYO SALAD

▲WF ▲GF   SERVES 3

There's a bit of Chopin in this classical dish. For ease of preparation, employ the Buddhist approach to vegetable chopping; breathe deeply and slowly whilst tapping into your innermost tranquillity.

500 g (1 lb 2 oz) chicken breast fillets

2 celery stalks, thinly sliced

1/2 red capsicum (pepper), seeds and membrane removed, diced

1/2 small red onion, chopped

1 granny smith apple, cored and chopped

1 large bunch English spinach leaves

Celtic sea salt and freshly ground black pepper

OMEGA-3 MAYO

1 organic egg

1 tablespoon freshly squeezed lemon juice

1/4 teaspoon Celtic sea salt

1 garlic clove, minced (optional)

125 ml (4 fl oz/1/2 cup) extra virgin olive oil

125 ml (4 fl oz/1/2 cup) flaxseed oil

Place the chicken breasts in a small, heavy-based saucepan. They should fit snugly in a single layer. Cover the chicken with broth or water and bring to the boil. Quickly reduce the heat to low so the liquid is barely a simmer. Partly cover and gently simmer for 10 minutes.

To make the mayonnaise, crack the egg into a food processor. Add the lemon juice, salt and garlic, if using, and process on low for a few seconds. With the motor still running on low, gradually add the olive oil – the slower the better. Keep the motor running and slowly add the flaxseed oil and continue to blend until the mixture is thick and creamy.

Place all the salad ingredients in a large bowl. Gently stir through the mayonnaise. Season to taste and serve.

NOTE: The mayo can be stored in the fridge in a sterilised, tightly-sealed jar for up to 7 days.

SWEET POTATO, CELERY AND APPLE

▲WF ▲DF ▲GF ▲VG   SERVES 3

The thing that makes this recipe amazing is the julienne technique used for the vegetables. Preparing the vegetables this way results in a highly delicate texture which is a delight to eat. Adding the mint gives it a punch and the dressing is a taste-bud explosion.

1 sweet potato, peeled and finely julienned

1 granny smith apple, cored and finely julienned

2 celery stalks, thinly sliced

3 tablespoons toasted sesame seeds

2 tablespoons thinly sliced mint leaves

DRESSING

2 tablespoons freshly squeezed lemon juice

1 tablespoon freshly grated ginger

2 tablespoons extra-virgin olive oil

1 garlic clove, minced

pinch of Celtic sea salt

freshly ground black pepper

To make the dressing, whisk all the ingredients together in a small bowl.

In a salad bowl, combine the sweet potato, apple, celery, sesame seeds and mint.

Drizzle over the dressing, season to taste, and serve.

▌SUPERCHARGED TIP▐

If you prefer a creamier dressing, blitz the ingredients with a hand blender until smooth.

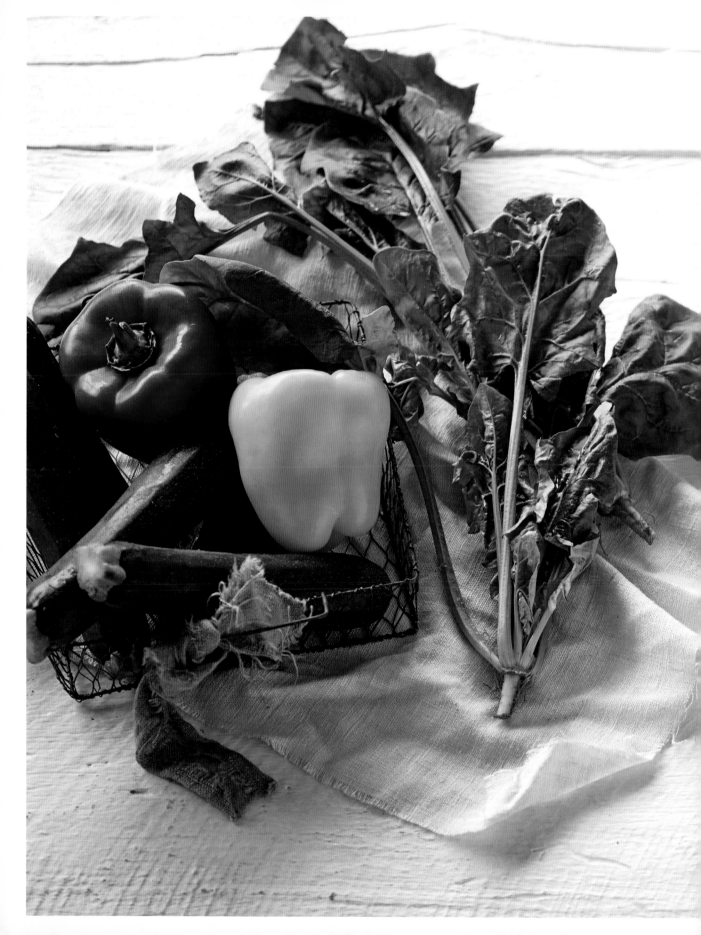

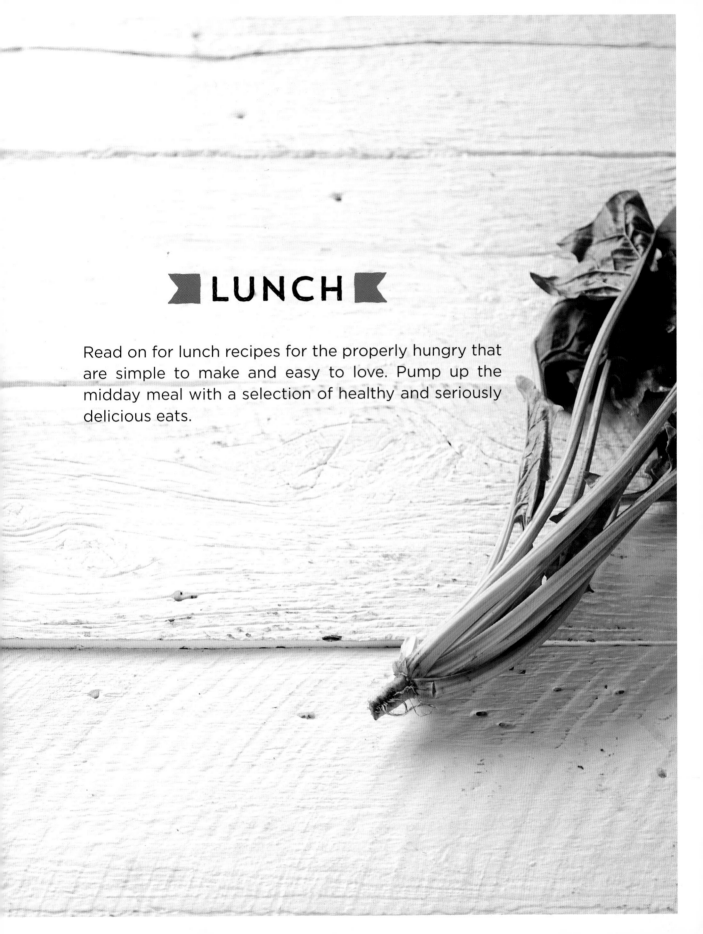

LUNCH

Read on for lunch recipes for the properly hungry that are simple to make and easy to love. Pump up the midday meal with a selection of healthy and seriously delicious eats.

WILD MUSHROOM, TOMATO AND SPINACH FRITTATA

▲WF ▲GF ▲SF   SERVES 6

I have never met a frittata that I didn't enjoy. What is so magnificent about frittatas is their flexibility and versatility. Just by changing the types of vegetables and herbs you use, you can create a new masterpiece every time.

9 organic eggs

large pinch of Celtic sea salt

freshly ground black pepper, to taste

1 small handful of basil leaves, roughly chopped

2 tablespoons extra virgin olive oil

1 small red onion, diced

2 garlic cloves, minced

90 g (3¹/4 oz/1 cup) sliced button mushrooms

4 large handfuls of baby English spinach leaves

80 g (2³/4 oz/²/3 cup) crumbled goat's cheese

Preheat the grill (broiler) to high.

Whisk the eggs, salt and pepper together in a large bowl. Add the basil and stir.

Heat the olive oil in a large, ovenproof frying pan over medium heat. Add the onion and cook, stirring occasionally, for 5 minutes, or until translucent. Add the garlic and mushrooms and sauté for a further 3 minutes. Add the spinach to the pan and cook for a couple of minutes, or until the spinach has wilted. Pour over the egg mixture, add the goat's cheese, and cook for 5 minutes.

Remove the saucepan from the heat and place it under the grill for 3 minutes, or until the top of the eggs are set. Remove from the grill and allow to cool slightly before dividing into slices and serving.

SARDINE AND ANCHOVY PIZZA

▲WF ▲GF ▲SF   MAKES 2 PIZZAS

I can't remember the last time I opened my pantry without discovering a tin of oily sustainable fish. Pizza is the perfect vehicle for sardines and anchovies, two of the most helpful inflammation-busting pantry standbys. Scatter them on top of a thin pizza base, pop in the oven and you are away.

PIZZA BASE

150 g (5¹/2 oz/1¹/2 cups) almond meal

2 organic eggs, beaten

2 tablespoons extra virgin olive oil

2 tablespoons nutritional yeast flakes

¹/2 teaspoon dried oregano

¹/2 teaspoon dried basil

2 garlic cloves, minced

¹/4 teaspoon Celtic sea salt

1 teaspoon apple cider vinegar

TOPPING

2 tablespoons additive-free tomato
    paste (concentrated purée)

100 g (3¹/2 oz) oven-roasted
    tomatoes (optional)

65 g (2¹/4 oz/²/3 cup) grated full-fat
    cheddar or 90 g (3¹/4 oz/³/4 cup)
    crumbled goat's cheese

160 g (5³/4 oz) tin sardines

5 anchovies

sprinkling of dulse flakes

Preheat the oven to 220°C (425°F/Gas 7) and lightly grease a pizza pan or large baking tray.

To make the pizza base, put all the ingredients in a large mixing bowl. Using your hands, mix well until you have a loose dough. If it feels too wet, add a bit more almond meal and work with your hands until smooth. Shape into a ball.

Divide the dough into two equal portions. Using a rolling pin, and working from the inside out in a clockwise motion, roll each portion out into a thin circle, about 15 cm (6 inches) in diameter. If you find the dough too sticky, add more almond meal. Place the two bases side by side on the prepared baking tray and cook in the oven for 10 minutes.

Remove from the oven and spread with the tomato paste, leaving a 1 cm (¹/2 inch) border of dough uncovered. Scatter the tomatoes (if using), cheese, sardines and anchovies over the top, and sprinkle with dulse flakes.

Return the pizzas to the oven for another 7–10 minutes, or until glistening and crispy. Serve hot.

▶HEALTH BENEFITS◀

The almond meal base is full of skin-boosting Vitamin E and protein.

HAZELNUT-CRUSTED WILD SALMON

▲WF ▲DF ▲GF ▲SF   SERVES 2

A foolproof dish for weekend lunch entertaining, crusted salmon makes good company and is simple and uncomplicated to create. Including the topping is crucial and ensures that as the salmon cooks the fish is self-basting, resulting in it being beautifully moist inside yet still bursting with flavour.

1 organic egg white, beaten

60 g (2¼ oz/½ cup) finely chopped
   toasted hazelnuts

1 teaspoon dried basil

2 wild-caught salmon steaks, skin on

large pinch of Celtic sea salt

freshly ground black pepper, to taste

25 g (1 oz/¼ cup) almond meal

2 tablespoons extra virgin olive oil

crunchy green salad, to serve

lemon cheeks, to serve

Preheat the oven to 200°C (400°F/Gas 6) and line a baking tray with baking paper.

Whisk the egg white and 1 tablespoon water together in a bowl.

In a separate, shallow bowl, combine the hazelnuts and basil.

Season the salmon fillets with salt and pepper. Coat the flesh side of the fillets with the almond meal, brush with the beaten egg white and then dip into the hazelnut and basil mixture.

Heat the olive oil in a large frying pan over medium heat and carefully lift the salmon into the pan, nut side down. Seal the salmon steaks for 2 minutes. Using a spatula, carefully turn the salmon and cook for a further 2–3 minutes.

Remove the salmon from the pan and place on the prepared baking tray. Cook in the oven for 10 minutes. Remove from the oven and serve with a crunchy green salad and lemon cheeks.

▶SUPERCHARGED TIP◀

Fifty per cent of the salmon we consume has been raised in fish farms. The salmon on these farms are often fed soy- and corn-based food, and fungicides are frequently used in the water, resulting in lower amounts of omega-3s. Farmed fish can look pale pink, so producers use a dye called canthaxanthin to strengthen the colour. Sound appetising? The solution: purchase wild-caught or organic farmed fish.

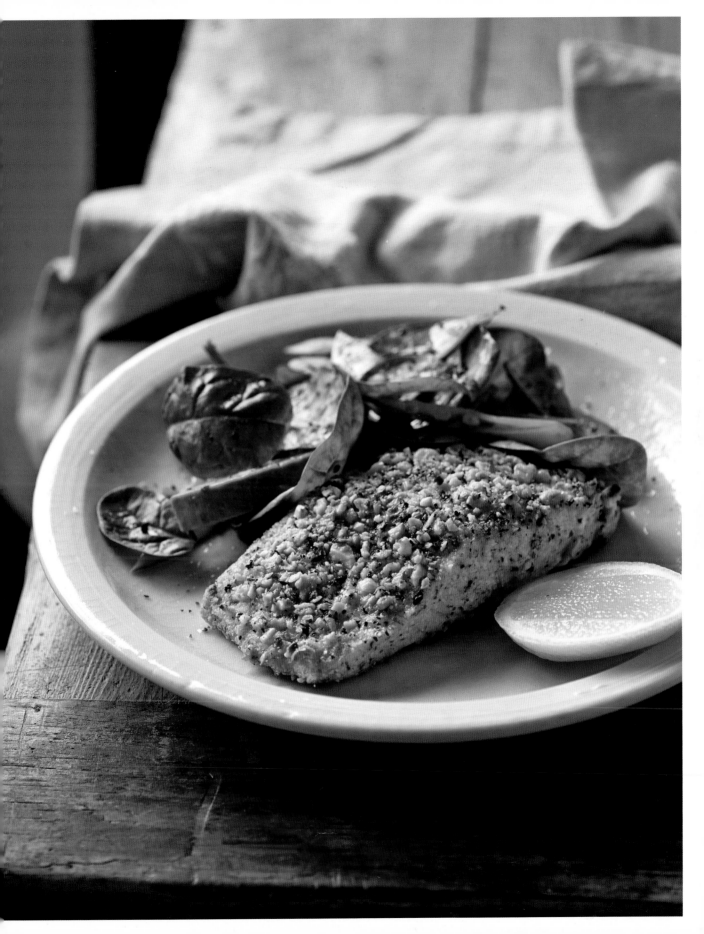

SUPERCHARGED OMELETTE

▲WF ▲GF ▲SF   SERVES 1

Ready in a matter of minutes and packed with goodness, this simple lunch omelette gives a little flavour kick with a host of wonderful nutrients to supercharge your afternoon.

1 tablespoon coconut oil, plus extra for greasing

1 green zucchini (courgette), sliced in thin pieces

2 tablespoons finely chopped red capsicum (pepper)

¼ teaspoon smoked paprika

1 tablespoon roughly chopped sun-dried tomatoes

2 large organic eggs

½ teaspoon finely grated lemon zest

Celtic sea salt

freshly ground black pepper

1 big handful of baby rocket (arugula) and baby English spinach mix

1 tablespoon finely grated vintage manchego (bitey Spanish sheep's cheese)

1 big handful of chopped coriander (cilantro) leaves and chives

Heat the coconut oil in a frying pan over high heat and sauté the zucchini and capsicum with the paprika for 7 minutes, stirring occasionally. Toss in the sun-dried tomatoes for added punch and cook for 5 minutes, or until lightly browned and fragrant. Reduce the heat to low.

Meanwhile, whisk the eggs lightly in a cup with the lemon zest, salt and pepper. In a second frying pan, add a little coconut oil over medium–low heat to grease the base then throw in the eggs. Make sure the heat is not too high or the omelette will burn. Cook until the omelette is slightly firm. Spread the vegetables over half the omelette and top with the spinach and rocket. When the eggs are set, use an egg flip to gently fold the half without toppings over the vegetables. Slide onto a serving plate, top with the coriander and chives and grated manchego.

Serve with a side salad drizzled with lemon and extra virgin olive oil, and another good pinch of salt and pepper to taste.

NOTE: This omelette also tastes wonderful with roasted pumpkin (winter squash) or sweet potato thrown in. A gluten-free mustard makes a wonderful condiment.

BROWN FRIED RICE

▲WF ▲DF ▲GF ▲SF   SERVES 4

Scrambled bits of egg, crispy brown rice, squashy peas and crunchy bacon combined in delicious tamari sauce. Who knew such a speedy dinner could taste so good?

1 tablespoon coconut oil

2 bacon slices, finely diced

2 spring onions (scallions), finely chopped

50 g (1³/4 oz/¹/3 cup) peas, fresh or frozen

40 g (1¹/2 oz) green beans, chopped into 2 cm (³/4 inch) pieces

1 carrot, finely diced

925 g (2 lb ¹/2 oz/5 cups) cooked and cooled brown rice (about 2 cups uncooked rice)

2 tablespoons wheat-free tamari

2 organic eggs, lightly beaten

Heat the coconut oil in a large frying pan over high heat until it is sizzling.

Add the bacon, spring onions, peas, beans and carrot and cook, stirring, for 7–10 minutes.

Add the rice and cook for a further 5 minutes, stirring occasionally (about once every 60 seconds). Add the tamari and cook, stirring for 2 minutes.

Move the ingredients to one side of the pan to make space for the eggs. Add the eggs, cook for 30 seconds, then scramble using a fork. Stir to mix the egg with the rest of the ingredients and serve.

▶SUPERCHARGED TIP◀

Use day-old cooked and cooled rice when frying, otherwise you will end up with a gluggy, sticky mess.

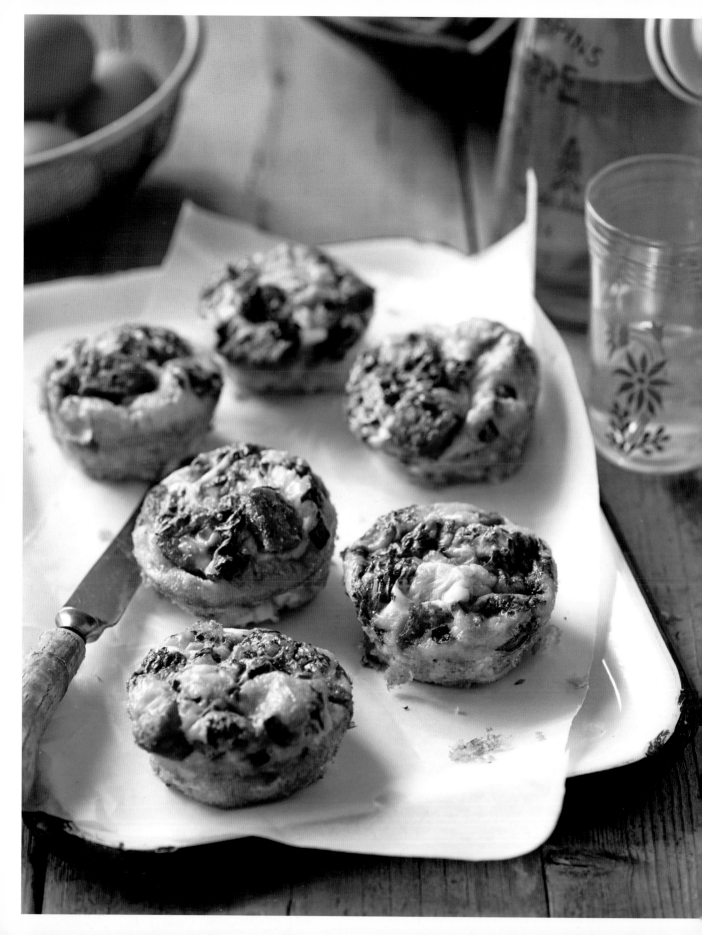

LAMB SAUSAGE AND BASIL EGG MUFFINS

▲WF ▲DF ▲GF ▲SF   MAKES 12

Give these a whirl and you'll never look at a fast-food sausage-and-egg muffin in the same way. Pack them into a lunchbox, parade them at picnics, or enjoy them sausage sizzling, just out of the oven beside a simple salad.

coconut oil, for greasing

12 organic eggs

4 large handfuls of basil leaves, chopped

Celtic sea salt and freshly ground black pepper, to taste

500 g (1 lb 2 oz) lamb sausages, cooked and chopped into bite-sized pieces

Preheat the oven to 180°C (350°F/Gas 4). Grease a 12-hole (80 ml/2½ fl oz/1/3 cup) muffin tin.

Crack the eggs into a large bowl, and whisk together. Add the basil and season.

Divide the sausage pieces evenly among the muffin holes. Pour over the eggs and cook in the oven for 15–20 minutes.

Remove from the oven and allow to cool in the tin, on a wire rack, for 5 minutes. Run a knife around the outside of each muffin to loosen, before turning them out of the tin.

They are delicious served warm or cold and will keep in a sealed container in the fridge for up to 4 days.

▶SUPERCHARGED TIP◀

These taste delicious cracked open and spread with butter. For a cheesy version, add 25 g (1 oz/1/4 cup) grated full-fat cheddar to the mix.

TUNA AND BROCCOLI MASHUP

▲WF ▲GF ▲SF   SERVES 2

What happens when you cross tuna and broccoli? A kind of magic occurs with these two nutritional superstars, making them a match made in foodie heaven. To make this dairy-free, substitute the parmesan for yeast flakes.

**2 broccoli heads and stems,
  roughly chopped**

80 ml (2¹/₂ fl oz/¹/₃ cup) almond milk

1 tablespoon extra virgin olive oil

**2 tablespoons freshly squeezed
  lemon juice**

1 teaspoon grated lemon zest

425 g (15 oz) tin tuna

large pinch of Celtic sea salt

freshly ground black pepper, to taste

**1 tablespoon grated parmesan or
  nutritional yeast flakes, plus extra
  to serve (optional)**

Place the broccoli in a steamer over a saucepan of gently simmering water and steam for 7–10 minutes, or until tender.

Remove the broccoli and place in a food processor with the almond milk. Blend for about 30 seconds. Add the remaining ingredients and blend until the mixture is smooth.

Serve sprinkled with extra parmesan or nutritional yeast flakes, if desired.

▶HEALTH BENEFITS◀

Say goodbye to orange peel thighs with broccoli, a detoxer's dream. Broccoli is loaded with Vitamins A and E, folate, calcium and iron and has a higher Vitamin C content than an orange. It contains an unusual combination of three phytonutrients: glucoraphanin, gluconasturtiin and glucobrassicin. Together these nutrients have a strong impact on our body's detoxification system, and can reduce the appearance of cellulite.

ZUCCHINI PASTA (ZOODLES) WITH BOLOGNESE

▲WF ▲DF ▲GF ▲SF   SERVES 2

Raw foodists have been singing their praises for years but perhaps you are new to zucchini noodles? You're in for a treat and once you've tried them you'll never return to ordinary noodles.

60 ml (2 fl oz/¼ cup) extra virgin olive oil

¼ onion, chopped

2 garlic cloves, minced

500 g (1 lb 2 oz) organic minced (ground) beef

4 tomatoes, chopped

125 ml (4 fl oz/½ cup) tomato passata (puréed tomatoes)

2 tablespoons sugar- and additive-free tomato paste (concentrated purée)

1½ teaspoons fresh or dried herbs, such as oregano, sage, basil and thyme

Celtic sea salt and freshly ground black pepper

2 tablespoons nutritional yeast flakes

fresh basil leaves, to serve

ZOODLES

1 celery stalk, thinly sliced

4 small zucchini (courgettes)

4 garlic cloves, sliced

2 tablespoons extra virgin olive oil

Heat the olive oil in a large frying pan over high heat. Add the onion and garlic and cook for 5 minutes, or until brown. Add the meat and cook for 10 minutes, or until tender. Add the tomatoes, passata, tomato paste and herbs, reduce the heat to low and simmer, stirring, for 15 minutes. Season to taste.

Meanwhile, make the pasta. Chop the celery and set aside.

Wash the zucchini and spiralise, using a vegetable spiraliser or spirooli machine.

Heat the olive oil in a frying pan over medium heat and cook the garlic for 5 minutes, or until soft. Add the zucchini and cook for 5 minutes.

Transfer to serving bowls, top with the bolognese and sprinkle with nutritional yeast flakes. Garnish with freshly picked basil leaves.

> **◥SUPERCHARGED TIP◤**
>
> You can also use a vegetable peeler to make ribbon strip zoodles. Chop the ends off your zucchini, then, holding the zucchini vertically in your hand, grate thin strips with your peeler. Rotate the zucchini as you grate so that the peeling is even, and stop once you hit the seeds.

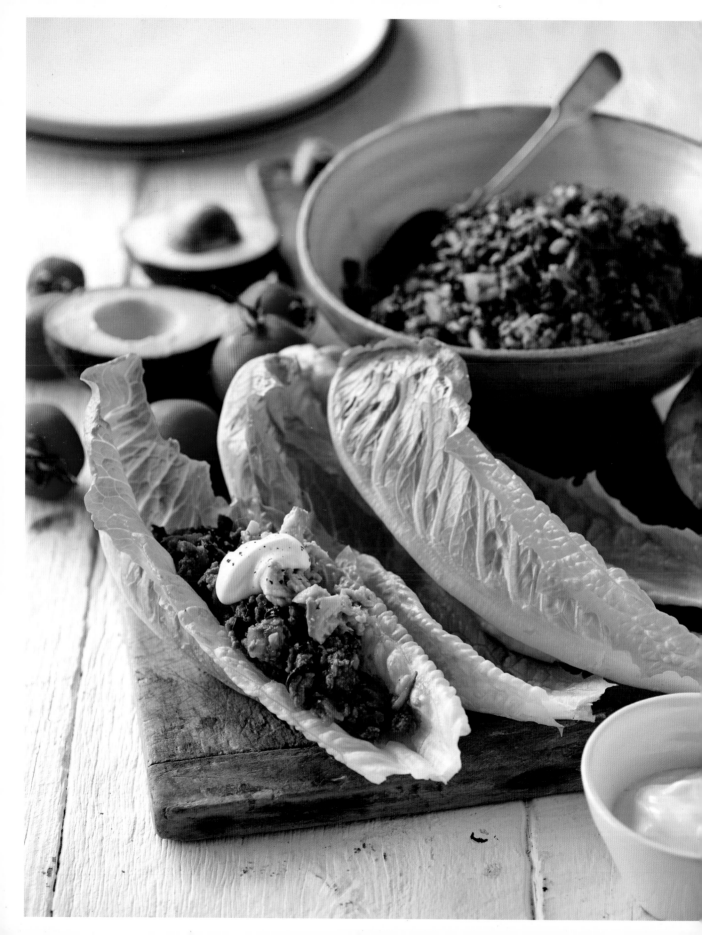

LETTUCE LEAF BURRITOS

▲WF ▲GF ▲SF   MAKES 12

Lettuce wraps are the latest trend in gluten-free burritos and homemade ones can be as healthy as all get out. These are perfect served with a dollop of avocado and a sprinkling of nutritional yeast flakes.

1 tablespoon extra virgin olive oil

1 red onion, diced

3 garlic cloves, minced

1 kg (2 lb 4 oz) organic minced (ground) beef

1 tablespoon additive-free tomato paste (concentrated purée)

1 bunch English spinach, leaves chopped

2 zucchini (courgettes), grated

3 tomatoes, diced

2 spring onions (scallions), thinly sliced

12 large whole cos (romaine) lettuce leaves

1 avocado, peeled, stone removed and mashed

130 g (4¹/₂ oz/¹/₂ cup) plain, full-fat additive-free Greek-style yoghurt

2 tablespoons nutritional yeast flakes

Heat the olive oil in a large, heavy-based frying pan and sauté the onion and garlic over medium heat for 5 minutes. Add the mince and cook, stirring occasionally and using a wooden spoon to break up any lumps, for 10 minutes. Add the tomato paste, spinach, zucchini, tomatoes and spring onions and stir for another 15 minutes. Season to taste.

Place a lettuce leaf on each plate. Divide the mince evenly over the top of the lettuce. Top with a spoonful of avocado and yoghurt, sprinkle with yeast flakes, wrap and enjoy.

FISH WITH MACADAMIA SALSA

▲WF ▲DF ▲GF ▲SF   SERVES 2

Cooking fish is an art that is simple to master. When cooked, the fish should flake with relative ease and be opaque in the centre. The salsa is what really takes this fish dish to the next level.

40 g (1½ oz/¼ cup) macadamia
  nuts, halved

1 tomato, chopped

1 avocado, peeled, stone removed and diced

3 tablespoons fresh coriander (cilantro)
  leaves, chopped

3 tablespoons flat-leaf (Italian) parsley,
  chopped

2 tablespoons extra virgin olive oil

2 garlic cloves, chopped

2 white-fleshed fish fillets

Place the macadamias, tomato, avocado, coriander and parsley in a bowl. Add a splash of the olive oil and set aside.

Add the remaining olive oil to a large frying pan over medium heat and sauté the garlic for 5 minutes, or until translucent. Add the fish and cook for 2 minutes. Carefully turn the fish, using a spatula, and cook for a further 2 minutes, or until cooked to your liking.

Transfer to serving plates and top with the salsa.

◗HEALTH BENEFITS◖

Macadamias are a healthy skin food, due to their natural monounsaturated fats, which contain oleic fatty acids and palmitoleic fatty acids. Palmitoleic acid is naturally present in our skin when we are young. It does decrease with age, so boosting your intake of macadamias will add moisture to your skin, leaving it supple.

CHICKEN AND SAGE BURGERS

▲WF ▲GF ▲SF   SERVES 5

These tasty burgers can be rustled up at a moment's notice when you don't feel like spending too much time in the kitchen. Chicken and sage are destined to be together with sage's aromatic personality working well to complement the chicken and aid in its digestion.

500 g (1 lb 2 oz) minced (ground) chicken

1/2 onion, diced

2 garlic cloves, minced

1 organic egg, lightly beaten

1 teaspoon sage

Celtic sea salt and freshly ground black
  pepper, to taste

1 tablespoon extra virgin olive oil

10 slices Chia and Flaxseed Loaf (see
  page 222), toasted

Omega-3 Mayo (see page 142), to serve

Combine the chicken, onion, garlic, egg and sage in a bowl and season with salt and pepper to taste.

Using your hands, divide the mixture into 5 patties.

Heat the olive oil in a large frying pan over medium heat and add the patties. Cook for 5 minutes, and then turn and cook for a further 5 minutes, or until cooked through.

Place each patty between 2 slices of Chia and Flaxseed Loaf, and serve with Omega-3 Mayo and cauliflower mash on the side.

▶ SUPERCHARGED TIP ◀

To make a delicious salad dressing, add fresh sage leaves to extra virgin olive oil and store in the refrigerator for up to 3 weeks. Sage leaves can also be frozen. All you need to do is take fresh sage sprigs, wash and pat them dry, remove the leaves from the stems, then pack them loosely in freezer bags. They can be frozen for up to 12 months. Freezing sage will intensify the flavour.

KEEN-WAH BURGERS

▲WF ▲DF ▲GF ▲SF   MAKES 10

Meatless burgers don't need to taste like cardboard or be hard to come by. A departure from the well-trodden soy-laden path, quinoa makes a subtle nutty and crunchy appearance. I just know these will become the burgers of your dreams.

1 tablespoon coconut oil

1 brown onion, chopped

225 g (8 oz/2^1/$_2$ cups) finely chopped
   button mushrooms

3 garlic cloves, minced

^{1}/$_2$ teaspoon dried oregano

^{1}/$_2$ teaspoon dried sage

1 organic egg

60 g (2^1/$_4$ oz/^{1}/$_2$ cup) finely chopped walnuts

35 g (1^1/$_4$ oz/^{1}/$_3$ cup) almond meal

1 tablespoon nutritional yeast flakes

1 tablespoon wheat-free tamari

100 g (3^1/$_2$ oz/^{1}/$_2$ cup) quinoa, cooked
   according to the packet instructions

large pinch of Celtic sea salt

freshly ground black pepper

Preheat the oven to 175°C (345°F/Gas 3–4) and line a baking tray with baking paper.

Heat the coconut oil in a large frying pan over medium heat and sauté the onion. Add the mushrooms, garlic, oregano and sage and cook for 5 minutes, stirring. Remove from the pan and set aside to cool.

Combine the egg, walnuts, almond meal, yeast flakes and tamari in a food processor and whizz for about 20 seconds. Add to the mushroom mixture along with the cooked quinoa, mix well and season, then, using your hands, shape the mixture into 10 equal patties.

Transfer to the baking tray and cook in the oven for 25 minutes.

Serve with a crispy salad or green beans.

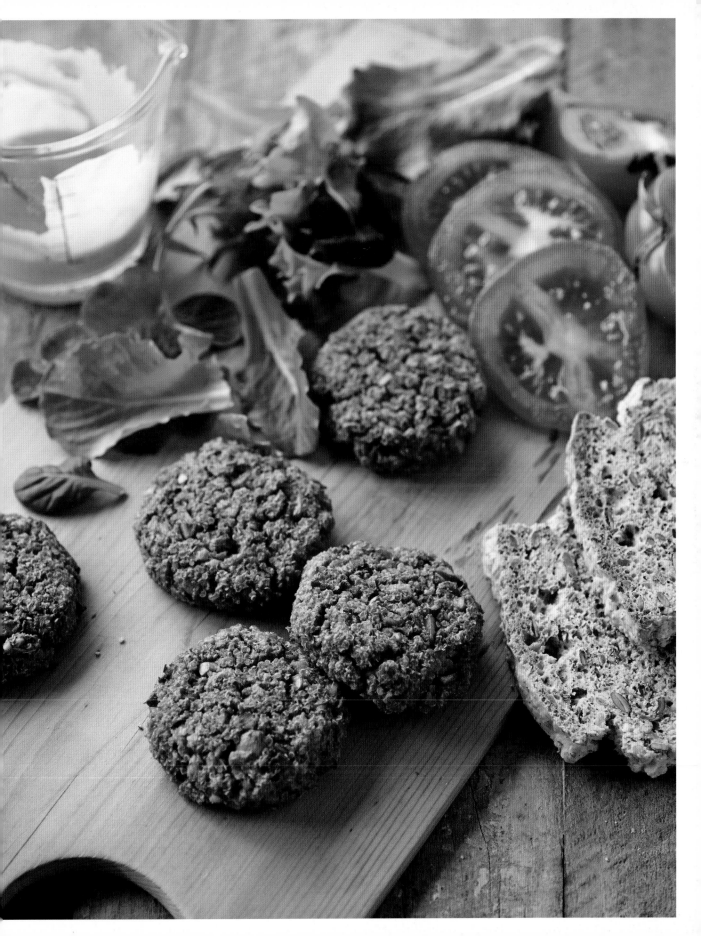

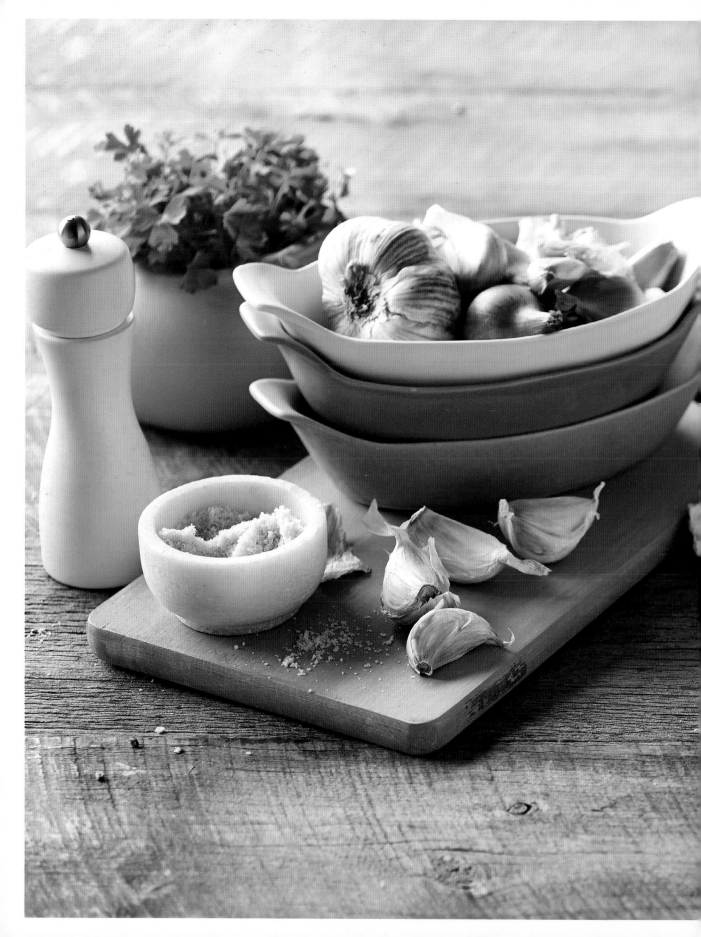

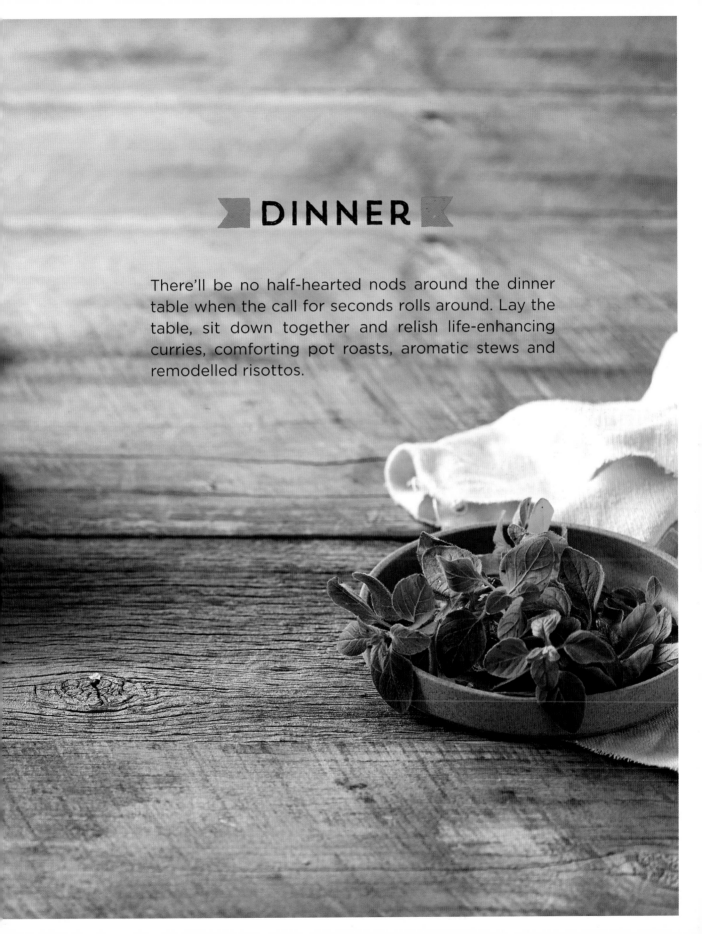

DINNER

There'll be no half-hearted nods around the dinner table when the call for seconds rolls around. Lay the table, sit down together and relish life-enhancing curries, comforting pot roasts, aromatic stews and remodelled risottos.

CHIA-GLAZED WILD SALMON

▲WF ▲DF ▲GF ▲SF   SERVES 4

This dish sounds like a fixture on a fancy restaurant menu, and that's exactly how it tastes – but it's extremely easy to make at home. For best results choose spanking fresh wild-caught Alaskan salmon. The marinade really brings the fish to life and cranks up the flavour.

4 pieces wild-caught salmon, skin on

MARINADE

125 ml (4 fl oz/1/2 cup) wheat-free tamari

1 tablespoon sesame oil

1 teaspoon freshly grated ginger

1 tablespoon additive-free dijon mustard

6 drops stevia liquid

4 spring onions (scallions), chopped

1 tablespoon chia seeds

greens, to serve

Preheat the oven to 200°C (400°F/Gas 6) and line a baking tray with baking paper.

Mix the marinade ingredients together in a large bowl. Add the salmon, cover and refrigerate for 20 minutes.

Place the salmon on the baking tray, skin side down, reserving the marinade. Bake in the oven for 20 minutes, or until the fish is cooked to your liking.

Dress with a couple of tablespoons of the reserved marinade and serve with your favourite greens.

▶**SUPERCHARGED TIP**◀

Serve over zoodles (zucchini noodles, see page 155) pan-fried in olive oil and garlic.

FISH AND VEGETABLE CURRY

▲WF ▲DF ▲GF ▲SF   SERVES 4

Curry is a sporty vehicle for omega-3-rich fish. This is a cinch to make and perfect for a quick and healthy mid-week dinner.

1 tablespoon coconut oil

1 brown onion, diced

2 garlic cloves, minced

2 tablespoons freshly grated ginger

400 ml (14 fl oz) additive-free coconut milk

2 tablespoons additive-free red curry paste

1 red capsicum (pepper), seeds and
   membrane removed, sliced

1/4 small white cabbage, thinly sliced

500 g (1 lb 2 oz) white-fleshed fish
   fillets, sliced

1 handful of coriander (cilantro) leaves,
   chopped, to serve

brown rice, to serve

Heat the coconut oil in a large saucepan over medium heat. Add the onion and garlic and stir around for 5 minutes, or until softened. Add the ginger, coconut milk and red curry paste and cook for 3 minutes, stirring until combined. Add the capsicum and cabbage, cover with a lid and simmer for 4–5 minutes. Add the fish and simmer for 5 minutes or until the fish is cooked through.

Serve with the coriander and brown rice.

BUCKWHEAT PASTA WITH FLAKED TROUT

▲WF ▲GF ▲SF   SERVES 2

This extremely quick, delicious pasta is wonderful for a simple dinner or fulfilling lunch. The fresh flavours of the trout and zesty lemon are superb with the earthiness of buckwheat pasta. Topped with rocket and chives for extra freshness, you'll discover a beautiful combination of textures and flavours.

1 generous-sized fresh trout fillet

125 g (4¹/2 oz) uncooked buckwheat pasta

2 organic egg yolks

zest and juice of 1 lemon

Celtic sea salt

freshly ground black pepper

1¹/2 tablespoons salted baby capers, rinsed

2 tablespoons extra virgin olive oil, plus extra, to serve

2 large handfuls of baby rocket (arugula)

2 tablespoons finely chopped chives

90 g (3¹/4 oz/³/4 cup) crumbled goat's cheese

Line a bamboo steamer with baking paper and steam the trout over a saucepan of gently simmering water for 5–6 minutes, or until the fish flakes when gently touched with a fork. Remove from the steamer, flake the flesh apart with a fork, removing any bones, and set aside.

Cook the pasta according to the packet instructions. Strain using a colander, reserving a little of the cooking water in the saucepan.

Return the pasta to the saucepan and quickly stir through the egg yolks, lemon juice and zest, and a generous pinch of Celtic sea salt and pepper. Gently stir through the flaked trout and capers and add the olive oil.

To serve, mix the rocket, chives, goat's cheese and extra olive oil, if desired, through the pasta and pop a wedge of lemon on the side. It's delicious served with a simple green salad.

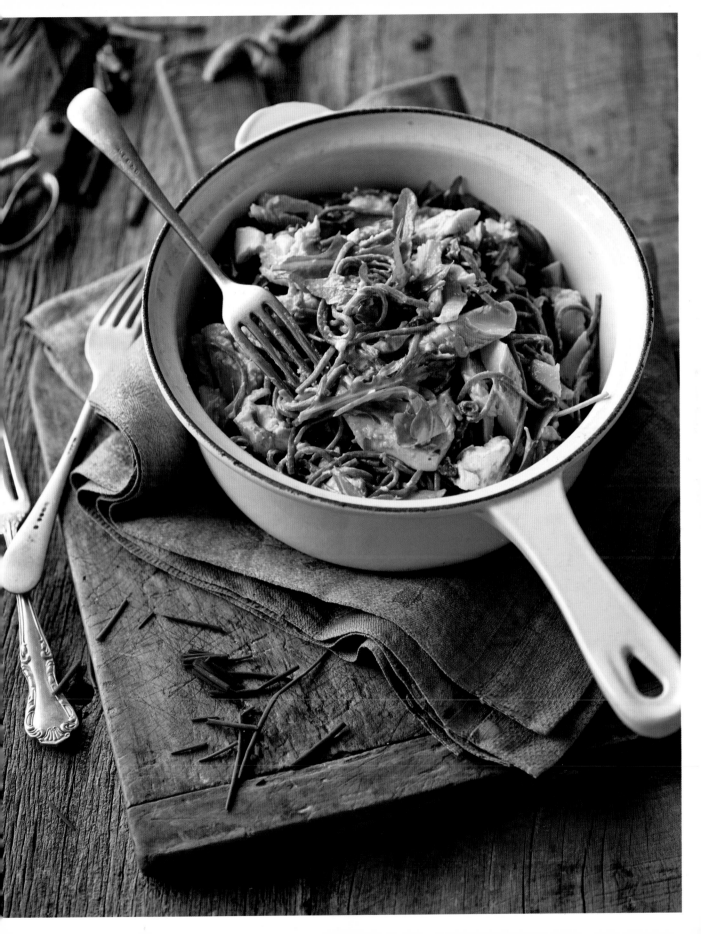

CHICKEN WITH KALE AND TURMERIC

▲WF ▲DF ▲GF ▲SF   SERVES 2–3

A chicken dinner for the soul, this quick eat will have you relishing in all the hallowed goodness that comes from the triple health benefits of chicken, kale and turmeric. It's a simple dish that can be ready on the dinner table in less than half an hour.

1 teaspoon ground turmeric

1 teaspoon ground cumin

1 small red chilli, finely chopped

1 teaspoon Celtic sea salt

2 garlic cloves, minced

500 g (1 lb 2 oz) skinless chicken breast fillets, diced

1 tablespoon coconut oil

1 small bunch kale leaves, washed and stems removed

1 red capsicum (pepper), seeds and membrane removed, diced

cooked quinoa, to serve

80 g (2³/₄ oz/¹/₂ cup) almonds, toasted, to serve

Combine the turmeric, cumin, chilli, sea salt and garlic in a medium bowl and mix well. Add the chicken and coat in the marinade.

Heat the coconut oil in a large frying pan over medium–high heat. Add the chicken and cook, stirring, for about 6 minutes. Add the kale leaves and capsicum and cook, stirring, for a further 10 minutes.

Serve with quinoa and top with toasted almonds.

BAKED WILD SALMON WITH PARSLEY AND WALNUTS

▲WF ▲DF ▲GF ▲SF   SERVES 2

Enjoy significant reductions in total and LDL cholesterol levels with this heart-healthy mixture of top-of-the-line good fats. Baking salmon is a very simple way to get delicious results without a lot of fuss and hardly any cleaning up. Who says eating healthy is hard work?

1 tablespoon coconut oil

2 wild-caught salmon fillets, skin on

2 tablespoons crushed walnuts

1 tablespoon flat-leaf (Italian) parsley, chopped

1/4 teaspoon Celtic sea salt (optional)

big squeeze of freshly squeezed lime juice, to serve

steamed green beans, to serve

Preheat the oven to 200°C (400°F/Gas 6) and lightly grease a baking tray with the coconut oil.

Place the salmon on the tray, skin side down. Sprinkle the walnuts, parsley and salt over the top. Transfer to the oven and cook for 12–15 minutes, or until the fish is cooked to your liking.

Remove from the oven, squeeze over the lime juice and serve with steamed green beans.

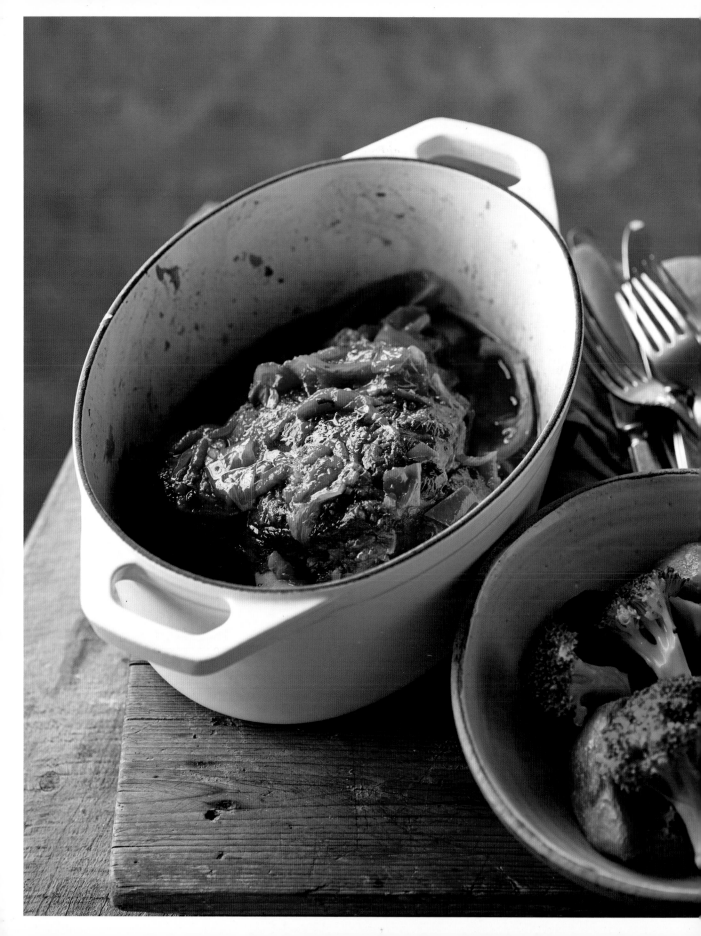

LAMB POT ROAST

▲WF ▲DF ▲GF ▲SF   SERVES 4–6

This meltingly tender hunter–gatherer dish is satisfyingly rich and virtually cooks itself. Pot roasting concentrates flavours and brings out the best in a leg of lamb. There'll be plenty of wrangling for places when you bring this dish to the table. The ideal accompaniments, which can be whipped up while the pot roast cooks and rests, are roasted turnips and steamed broccoli.

2 kg (4 lb 8 oz) leg of lamb

4 garlic cloves, sliced

1 tablespoon basil leaves

1 tablespoon extra virgin olive oil

1 brown onion, cut into wedges

500 ml (17 fl oz/2 cups) homemade
   additive-free chicken stock

1 tablespoon apple cider vinegar

80 ml (2½ fl oz/⅓ cup) freshly squeezed
   lemon juice

1 large red capsicum (pepper), seeds and
   membrane removed, roughly chopped

Celtic sea salt and freshly ground
   black pepper

2 lemon wedges

2 tablespoons dried oregano

2 tablespoons flat-leaf (Italian)
   parsley, chopped

roasted turnips and steamed broccoli,
   to serve

Make four incisions in the lamb with a sharp knife, inserting the garlic and basil into the incisions.

Heat the olive oil in a heavy-based flameproof casserole dish over medium–high heat and seal the lamb for 3 minutes on each side, or until browned. Remove the lamb from the dish and set aside.

Add the onion to the casserole dish and cook for 4 minutes. Stir in the stock, vinegar and lemon juice. Return the lamb and add the capsicum to the casserole dish and season with salt and pepper. Reduce the heat to very low and simmer, covered, for 1 hour. Turn the lamb and return to the heat for another hour. Add the lemon wedges and oregano, return to the heat and simmer for a further 30 minutes.

Remove from the heat, sprinkle with the parsley and serve with roasted turnips and steamed broccoli.

JOLLY GOOD BUTTER CHICKEN

▲WF ▲GF   SERVES 4–6

Kim Cotton, who blogs at www.spiritedmama.com, is part of the sisterhood and loves to come around for a Jolly Good Butter Chicken on a Friday night. It's the ultimate comfort food that sees many through the trials and tribulations of love and life. This recipe is a great way to indulge in health-promoting spices.

1 tablespoon sesame oil

1 kg (2 lb 4 oz) free-range chicken breast fillets, thickly sliced

70 g (2¹⁄₂ oz) unsalted butter

1 teaspoon garam masala

1 cinnamon stick

10 cardamom pods

1 teaspoon sweet paprika

1 teaspoon ground cumin (optional)

1 teaspoon ground chilli (optional)

400 g (14 oz) tin chopped tomatoes

1 tablespoon sugar- and additive-free tomato paste (concentrated purée)

400 ml (14 oz) additive-free coconut milk

1 ripe banana, sliced

1 teaspoon shredded coconut

370 g (12³⁄₄ oz/2 cups) steamed brown rice

1 Lebanese (short) cucumber, diced and chilled

1 dollop of mango chutney (optional)

Place a large heavy-based saucepan over high heat and add the sesame oil. Cook the chicken in two batches, turning regularly for about 5 minutes or until browned. Remove from the pan and set aside while you cook the remaining chicken. Remove it from the pan.

Reduce the heat a little and add the butter. When the butter has melted add the spices and cook, stirring, for 4–5 minutes until fragrant.

Return the chicken to the pan, along with the tomatoes and tomato paste. Stir and simmer for about 20 minutes.

Turn down the heat to low and stir in the coconut milk. Simmer for about 5 minutes.

Mix the banana and coconut together in a small bowl.

Serve the butter chicken with the brown rice, chilled cucumber, banana with coconut and some mango chutney, if desired.

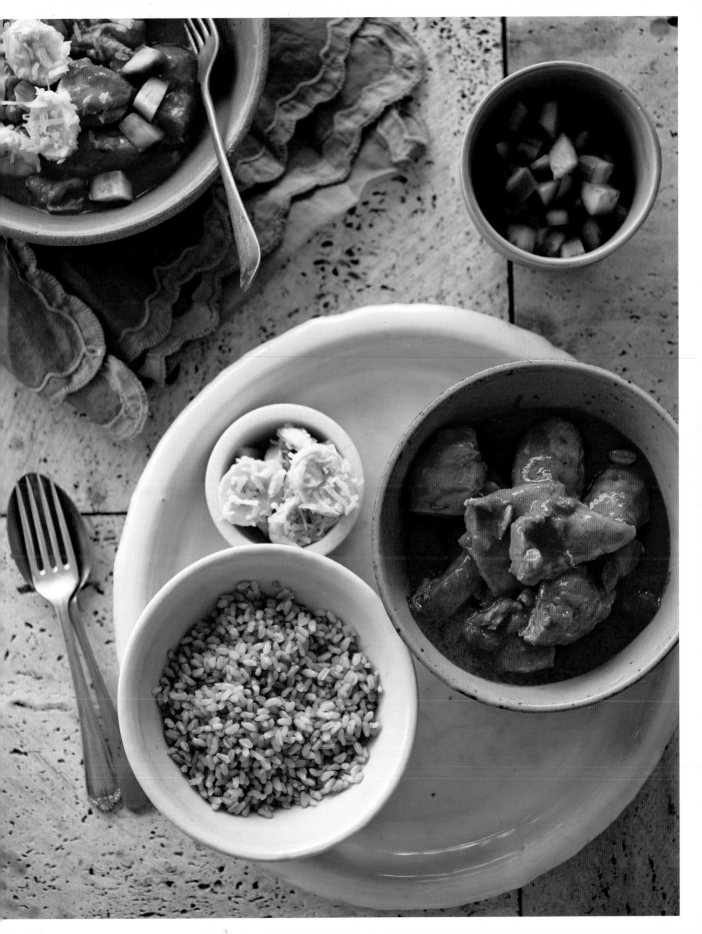

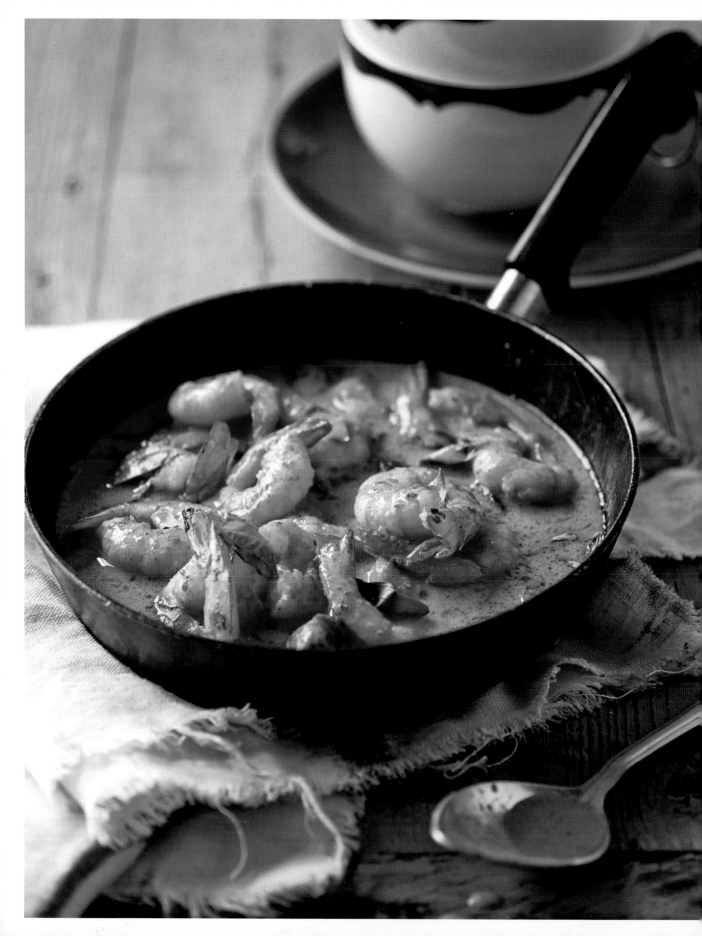

STIR-FRIED RED PRAWNS

▲WF ▲DF ▲GF ▲SF   SERVES 4

This is fast and easy and so good for you. Prawns contain a natural pink pigment astaxanthin, a powerful antioxidant which protects skin against sun damage and improves its elasticity. It even helps to improve uneven skin tone, leaving you with a youthful healthy glow. Think pink. Eat more prawns.

500 g (1 lb 2 oz) peeled and deveined raw prawns (shrimp)

2 tablespoons red curry paste

2 garlic cloves, minced

1 teaspoon freshly grated ginger

juice of 1 lime

1 tablespoon coconut oil

400 ml (14 fl oz) additive-free coconut milk

1 handful of basil leaves

Asian greens, to serve

Combine the prawns, red curry paste, garlic, ginger and lime juice in a large bowl. Cover and refrigerate for 1 hour.

Remove the prawns from the fridge. Heat the coconut oil in a large frying pan over medium–high heat. Add the prawns and sauté for a couple of minutes. Pour in the coconut milk and add the basil and cook for a further minute.

Serve immediately on a bed of Asian greens.

MUSHROOM AND ALMOND LOAF

▲WF ▲DF ▲GF ▲SF ▲VG   SERVES 4–6

This hearty meaty loaf concocted by my lovely friend Holly McBride is a wonderful winter warmer. Feel free to experiment with your favourite mushrooms or use a combination. I adore mushrooms, and their anti-inflammatory status and immune-boosting properties have long been recognised and documented. Contemporary studies demonstrate what our ancestors knew a long time ago – mushrooms are a potent and powerful medicine and have such potential for restoring health and wellness.

80 g (2³/₄ oz/¹/₂ cup) buckwheat

1 tablespoon extra virgin olive oil

2 garlic cloves, minced

200 g (7 oz) button mushrooms, sliced

200 g (7 oz/1¹/₃ cups) chopped almonds

1 leek (about 200 g/7 oz), white part only, trimmed, washed and chopped

2 teaspoons of Italian dried herbs (or a mixture of thyme and rosemary)

Celtic sea salt and freshly ground black pepper

4 organic eggs

125 ml (4 fl oz/¹/₂ cup) almond milk

Cook the buckwheat according to the packet instructions and set aside to cool.

Preheat the oven to 200°C (400°F/Gas 6) and grease and line a 20 x 9 cm (8 x 3¹/₂ inch) loaf (bar) tin.

Heat the olive oil in a frying pan over medium–high heat and sauté the garlic, mushrooms, almonds and leek for 5 minutes. Add the herbs, salt and pepper. Cook for 10 minutes, stirring occasionally, then remove from the pan and set aside.

Meanwhile, in a separate bowl, mix the eggs, almond milk and buckwheat and season with salt and pepper. Stir in the mushroom and almond mixture.

Pour the mixture into the prepared tin. Bake in the oven for 45 minutes or until skewer inserted into the centre of the loaf comes out clean.

CHICKEN CASSEROLE WITH MACADAMIA AND BASIL

▲WF ▲DF ▲GF ▲SF   SERVES 4

60 ml (2 fl oz/¼ cup) extra virgin olive oil

500 g (1 lb 2 oz) chicken thigh fillets

1 brown onion, diced

4 garlic cloves, minced

1 yellow capsicum (pepper), seeds
  and membrane removed, diced

1 teaspoon Celtic sea salt

freshly ground black pepper

500 ml (17 fl oz/2 cups) chicken stock

135 g (4¾ oz/1 cup) ground macadamias

1½ tablespoons ground turmeric

2 tablespoons freshly squeezed lemon juice

1 teaspoon grated lemon zest

2 tablespoons nutritional yeast flakes

1 large handful of basil leaves, chopped

brown rice, to serve

Heat 1 tablespoon of the olive oil in a large heavy-based saucepan or flameproof casserole dish over medium–high heat. Add the chicken and cook for 4 minutes on each side. Remove from the pan and set aside. Add the remaining oil to the pan and sauté the onion, garlic and capsicum for 5 minutes, or until brown.

Return the chicken to the pan. Season with salt and pepper then add the stock and macadamias. Bring to the boil then reduce the heat and simmer for 5 minutes. Add the turmeric, lemon juice and lemon zest and stir. Reduce the heat, cover, and cook over low heat for 40 minutes, stirring occasionally.

To serve, stir in the yeast flakes and sprinkle with the basil. Serve with brown rice.

▶HEALTH BENEFITS◀

Basil is packed with iron and magnesium, which helps improve the blood circulation in the body and the essential oil eugenol, which provides anti-inflammatory effects similar to those of aspirin or ibuprofen.

COCONUT LAMB WITH CAULIFLOWER RICE

▲WF ▲DF ▲GF ▲SF   SERVES 4

Your nose will twitch at the first delicious whiff and your taste buds will be tickled by this new take on a fundamental classic stew. Substitute carbohydrate-heavy rice with delicious and nutritious cauliflower and you'll be left without the lingering sluggishness rice often brings.

1 tablespoon coconut oil

1/2 brown onion, diced

2 garlic cloves, sliced

600 g (1 lb 5 oz) lamb, cubed

4 tomatoes, diced

2 turnips, diced

800 ml (28 fl oz) additive-free coconut milk

2 zucchini (courgettes), halved lengthways
  and sliced

pinch of Celtic sea salt and freshly ground
  black pepper, to taste

3 tablespoons chopped coriander
  (cilantro) leaves

CAULIFLOWER RICE

1 small head of cauliflower

pinch of Celtic sea salt

freshly ground black pepper

2 tablespoons extra virgin olive oil

2 garlic cloves, minced

Melt the coconut oil in a heavy-based saucepan over medium heat. Add the onion and garlic and cook for 5–7 minutes, or until the onions are translucent. Add the lamb and sear before adding the tomatoes, turnips and coconut milk to the pan. Simmer, uncovered, for 45 minutes.

Meanwhile, make the cauliflower rice. Cut the core out of the cauliflower and discard. Place the cauliflower florets in a food processor and pulse until it is a fine grain. Season with salt and pepper.

Heat the olive oil in a frying pan over medium–high heat and add the garlic. Cook for 5 minutes. Add the cauliflower and cook for 5–7 minutes, or until al dente.

Add the zucchini to the pan with the lamb and continue to cook for a further 5 minutes.

Season with salt and pepper top with the coriander and serve over the cauliflower rice.

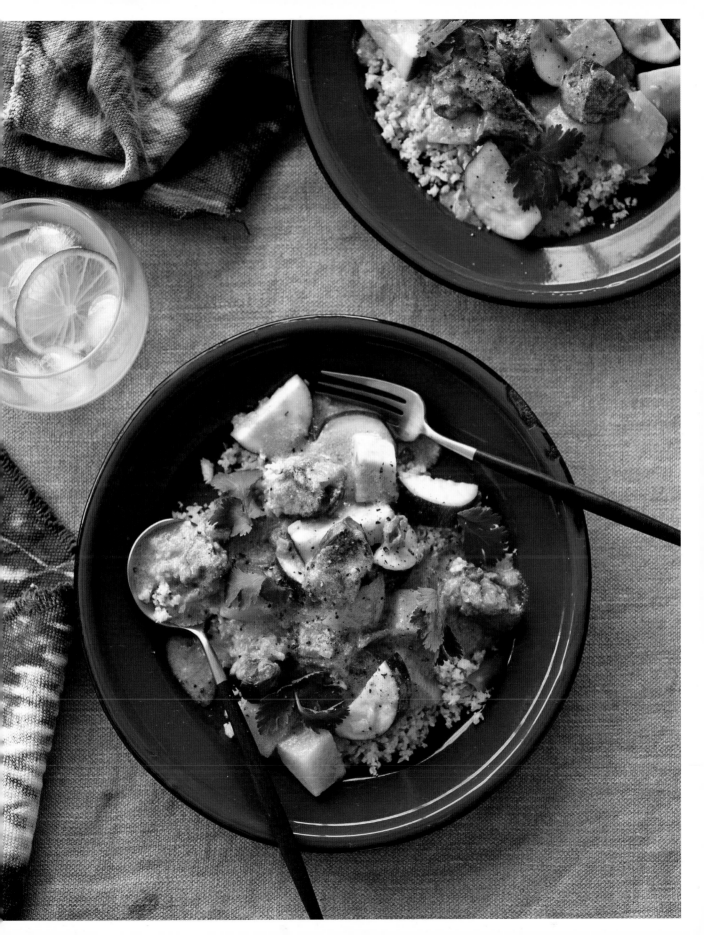

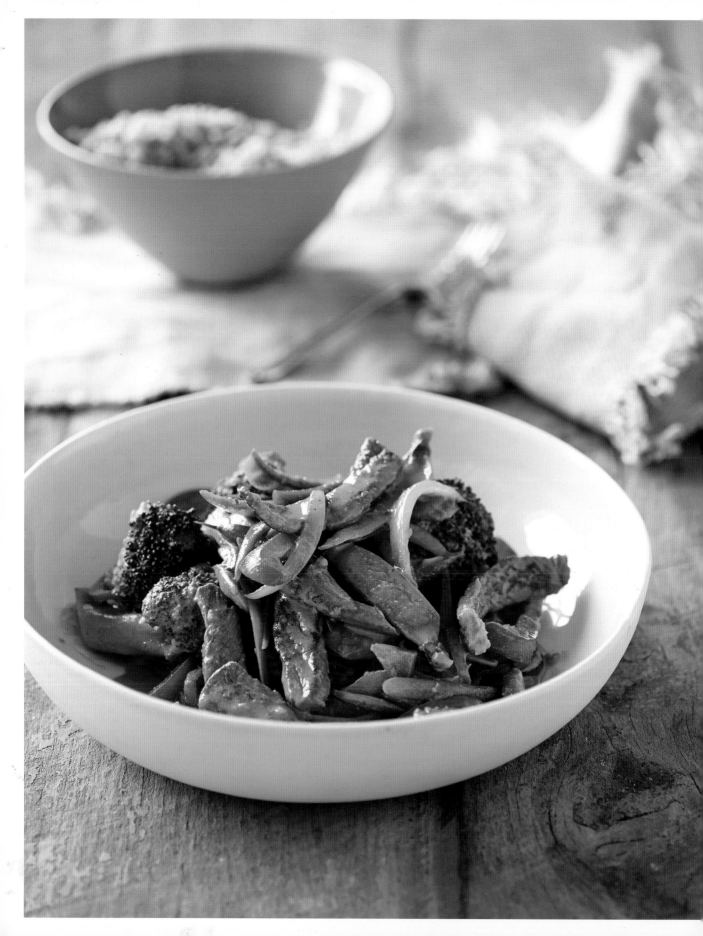

STIR-FRIED GINGER BEEF

▲WF ▲DF ▲GF ▲SF   SERVES 4

Behold the idiot-proof dinner. You'll be heaping this onto your spoon and cramming it into your mouth in just a very short space of time.

2 tablespoons coconut oil

1 brown onion, sliced

2 garlic cloves, minced

1/2 red capsicum (pepper), seeds and membrane removed, sliced

500 g (1 lb 2 oz) beef, cut into very thin strips

1 teaspoon ground turmeric

2 tablespoons freshly squeezed lemon juice

2 teaspoons freshly grated ginger

2 tablespoons wheat-free tamari

2 tablespoons tahini

1 tablespoon apple cider vinegar

120 g (4 1/4 oz/2 cups) broccoli florets

125 g (4 1/2 oz) green beans, roughly chopped

100 g (3 1/2 oz) snow peas (mangetout), sliced on the diagonal

Celtic sea salt and freshly ground black pepper, to taste

brown rice, to serve

Put the coconut oil in a large frying pan over medium–high heat. Add the onion, garlic and capsicum and sauté for 5–7 minutes. Add the beef and cook, stirring, for 5 minutes. Add the turmeric, lemon juice, ginger, tamari, tahini and vinegar. Cook, stirring, for 1 minute. Add the broccoli, beans and snow peas to the pan. Cook over medium heat for 12–15 minutes, or until the vegetables are tender.

Season with salt and pepper to taste and serve with brown rice.

▶HEALTH BENEFITS◀

Ginger contains potent anti-inflammatory compounds called gingerols. These substances, when consumed regularly, can help many people who are suffering from inflammatory conditions such as osteoarthritis or rheumatoid arthritis.

HERB-CRUSTED FISH WITH RUBY QUINOA

▲WF ▲DF ▲GF ▲SF   SERVES 2

If you need an easy fish dish for your weekly repertoire, this herb-crusted fish is as virtuous as it is simple. What more could you wish for?

45 g (1½ oz/⅓ cup) buckwheat flour

Celtic sea salt and freshly ground black pepper, to taste

1 tablespoon mixed dried herbs, such as basil, oregano, chives and sage

125 ml (4 fl oz/½ cup) homemade almond or cashew milk

2 white-fleshed fish, such as whiting, John Dory or silver bream

coconut oil, for pan-frying

QUINOA

100 g (3½ oz/½ cup) royal red quinoa

2 tablespoons slivered almonds

½ cup mixed herbs, such as dill, flat-leaf (Italian) parsley, coriander (cilantro), mint

30 g (1 oz/¼ cup) roughly chopped walnuts

grated lemon zest

4 large handfuls of baby English spinach leaves, roughly chopped

extra virgin olive oil, to drizzle

1 handful of baby rocket (arugula), to garnish (optional)

lemon wedges, to serve (optional)

Place the quinoa and 250 ml (9 fl oz/1 cup) filtered water in a saucepan with a pinch of sea salt. Bring to the boil, cover, reduce the heat to medium–low and cook for 15 minutes. Lift the lid, fluff the quinoa with a fork and set aside.

In a small frying pan, lightly toss the slivered almonds over high heat until toasty and golden brown. Set aside.

Mix the buckwheat flour with the salt and pepper and dried herbs in a shallow bowl. Put the nut milk in a separate bowl.

Dip the fish into the nut milk and then coat with the seasoned and herbed flour.

Heat the coconut oil in a frying pan over high heat and add the fish, cooking for 4 minutes (turning once), until the fish flakes when touched lightly with a fork and it is slightly golden, with crisped edges.

Meanwhile, in your favourite salad bowl, toss the quinoa, fresh herbs, almonds, walnuts, lemon zest, salt, pepper and baby English spinach together. Mix well and drizzle generously with olive oil.

Serve the fish with the baby rocket and lemon wedges, if using, and quinoa salad on the side.

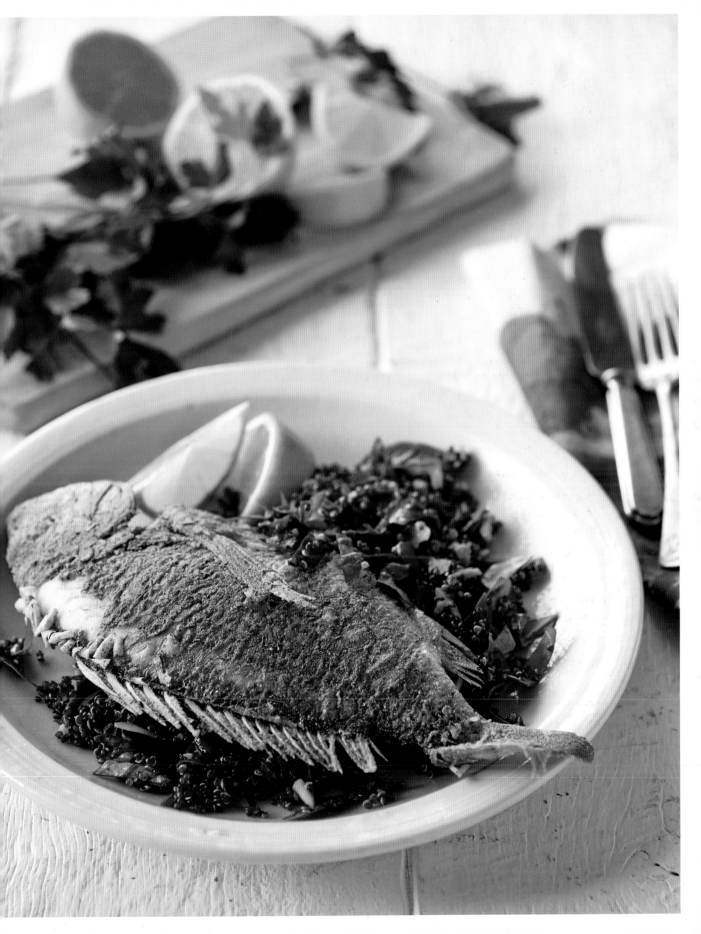

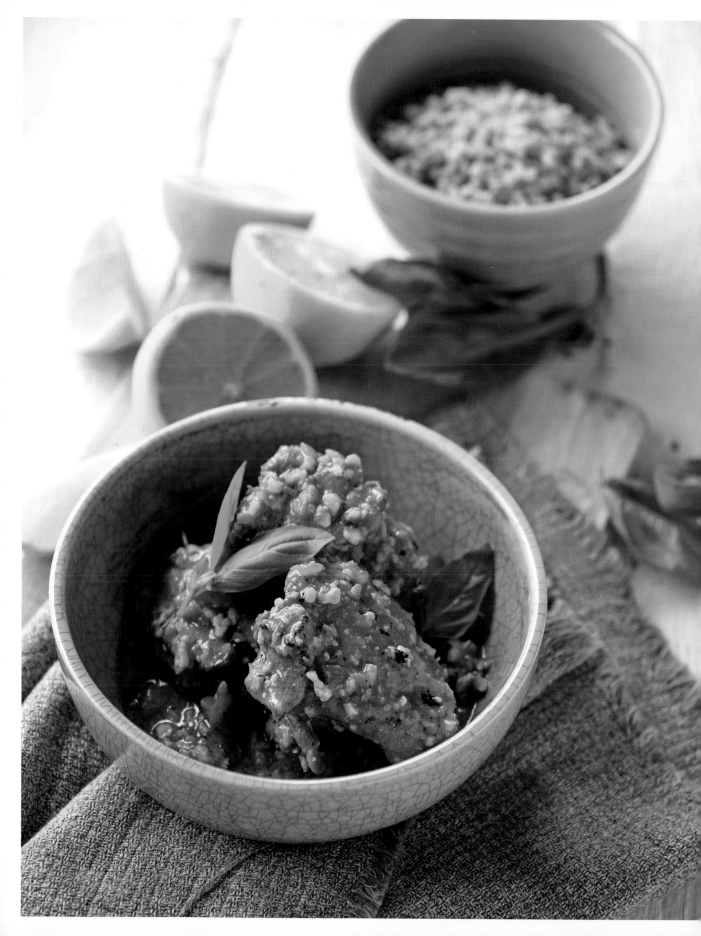

SWEET PISTACHIO CHICKEN

▲WF ▲DF ▲GF ▲SF   SERVES 4

How sweet it is for your body to be loved by this dish. So pretty and heart-achingly good for you. Pistachios are an excellent source of Vitamin E, a powerful lipid-soluble antioxidant which is essential for maintaining the integrity of cell membranes and offering your skin protection from harmful radicals.

60 ml (2 fl oz/¼ cup) extra virgin olive oil

1 tablespoon thyme

1 teaspoon Celtic sea salt

freshly ground black pepper, to taste

4 chicken breast fillets

2 garlic cloves, sliced

80 ml (2½ fl oz/⅓ cup) apple cider vinegar

2 tablespoons rice malt syrup, or 6 drops stevia liquid

125 ml (4 fl oz/½ cup) chicken stock or filtered water

65 g (2¼ oz/½ cup) chopped pistachios

Combine 1 tablespoon of the olive oil, the thyme, salt and pepper in a bowl. Rub the mixture into the chicken.

Heat 1 tablespoon of the oil in a heavy-based frying pan over medium heat and sauté the garlic for 5 minutes. Add the chicken and cook for 15–20 minutes, turning regularly.

Remove the chicken from the pan, set aside in a serving dish and keep warm.

Meanwhile, put the vinegar and remaining oil in a saucepan and cook for 1 minute, stirring constantly. Add the rice malt syrup or stevia and the stock to the pan and simmer for about 10 minutes, until the sauce starts to thicken. Add the pistachios and cook for 1 minute.

Pour the sauce over the chicken and serve.

BUCKWHEAT RISOTTO WITH SPINACH AND MUSHROOM

▲WF ▲DF ▲GF ▲SF ▲VG   SERVES 4

After some alterations to an ordinary risotto recipe – the first being to scrap the signature ingredient arborio rice – I have created a medicinal masterpiece. Gasp-worthily controversial to some, I've replaced the arborio with buckwheat and I am pleased to say that it works really well.

390 g (13³/₄ oz/2 cups) buckwheat

1 tablespoon extra virgin olive oil

1 onion, chopped

3 garlic cloves, minced

180 g (6¹/₄ oz/2 cups) sliced button mushrooms

500 ml (17 fl oz/2 cups) vegetable stock

1 teaspoon grated lemon zest

2 tablespoons freshly squeezed lemon juice

2 tablespoons apple cider vinegar

5 bunches English spinach, leaves shredded

2 tablespoons chopped spring onion (scallion)

¹/₂ teaspoon Celtic sea salt

80 ml (2¹/₂ fl oz/¹/₃ cup) additive-free coconut milk

2 tablespoons nutritional yeast flakes

Rinse the buckwheat in a sieve under running water and set aside.

Add the olive oil to a frying pan over medium heat and sauté the onion and garlic for 5 minutes, or until the onion is translucent. Add the buckwheat to the pan and stir to coat. Add the mushrooms and half the stock, the lemon zest and juice and vinegar and bring to the boil, stirring constantly. Reduce the heat and simmer for 10–12 minutes, or until all the liquid has been absorbed. Add the remaining stock and cook for a further 10–12 minutes, or until the stock has been absorbed and the buckwheat is tender.

Stir in the spinach and spring onion and season to taste. Add the coconut milk and cook for a further 3 minutes.

Serve sprinkled with the yeast flakes.

▶HEALTH BENEFITS◀

Buckwheat boasts a myriad of health benefits, containing the eight essential amino acids and several minerals including zinc, iron, manganese, potassium, phosphorus, copper and magnesium, and it is high in B-group vitamins that are essential to energy production and the optimum functioning of your digestive system.

IRISH STEW

▲WF ▲GF ▲SF   SERVES 6–8

Here's a stew that Irish mammys would be proud to call their own. It needs a couple of hours in the oven to nail the essence but it's well worth every lingering minute. Browning the meat initially boosts the flavour of the entire dish and red capsicum adds a touch of sweetness.

80 ml (2½ fl oz/⅓ cup) extra virgin olive oil

1 kg (2 lb 4 oz) deboned lamb shoulder, cut into 5 cm (2 inch) pieces

1 brown onion, chopped

6 garlic cloves, minced

1 leek, white part only, trimmed, washed and chopped

pinch of Celtic sea salt

freshly ground black pepper

1 tablespoon chopped rosemary leaves

2 tablespoons apple cider vinegar

2 teaspoons sweet paprika

1 red capsicum (pepper), seeds and membrane removed, cut into 1 cm (½ inch) strips

400 g (14 oz) additive-free tin chopped tomatoes

2 tablespoons chopped parsley

1 bay leaf

375 ml (13 fl oz/1½ cups) homemade chicken stock

CAULIFLOWER MASH

1 cauliflower, cut into florets

20 g (¾ oz) organic unsalted butter

1 tablespoon nutritional yeast flakes

Preheat the oven to 180°C (350°F/Gas 4).

In a heavy-based frying pan, heat 2 tablespoons of the olive oil. Add the meat in two batches, browning on all sides. Remove from the pan and set aside.

In a flameproof casserole dish, heat the remaining 2 tablespoons of oil. Add the onion, garlic and leek and sauté for 5–7 minutes, or until the vegetables are translucent. Add the lamb and all the remaining ingredients, adding the stock last.

Cover with a lid and cook in the oven for 2 hours, checking occasionally to ensure that it is not drying out – if it is, add more stock or filtered water.

To make the cauliflower mash, put the florets in a bamboo steamer over a saucepan of simmering water and cook, covered, for 15–20 minutes, or until tender – the florets can be verging on soft, but shouldn't be falling apart.

Transfer the cauliflower to a blender or food processor and add the butter, yeast flakes, a pinch of sea salt and a few grinds of black pepper. Blend until smooth.

Serve the stew piping hot over the cauliflower mash.

▶ **SUPERCHARGED TIP** ◀

For a thicker, chunkier stew, I like to throw in a diced turnip prior to putting it in the oven.

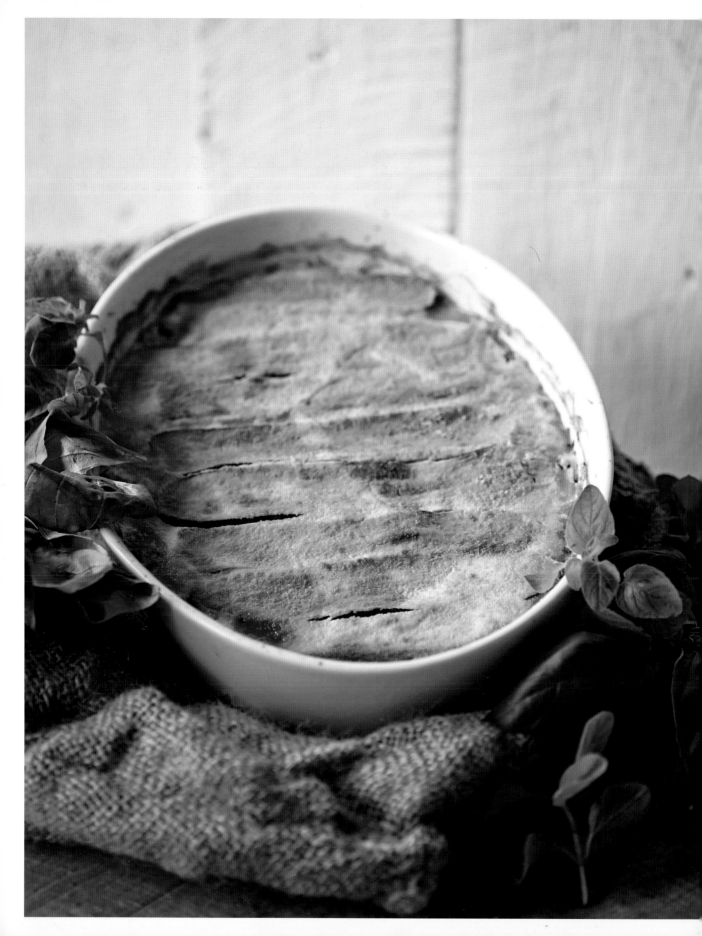

SUPERCHARGED LASAGNE

▲WF ▲GF ▲SF　　　SERVES 4

Making a concerted effort to eat more vegetables and fewer processed foods will have an ahhh-mazing effect on your body. Even if you feel the irresistible lure of comfort food, including a couple of healthy swap-outs, like using zucchini in place of pasta and adding yoghurt instead of white sauce means you can still enjoy a wonderfully healthy and filling meal such as this scrumptious supercharged lasagne.

unsalted butter, for greasing

60 ml (2 fl oz/1/4 cup) extra virgin olive oil

3 small zucchini (courgettes), sliced
　lengthways into 5 mm (1/4 inch) pieces

1/4 onion, chopped

2 garlic cloves, minced

500 g (1 lb 2 oz) organic minced
　(ground) beef

4 tomatoes, chopped

125 ml (4 fl oz/1/2 cup) tomato passata
　(puréed tomatoes)

2 tablespoons sugar- and additive-free
　tomato paste (concentrated purée)

11/2 teaspoons fresh or dried herbs,
　such as oregano, sage, basil and thyme

Celtic sea salt and freshly ground
　black pepper

200 g (7 oz/3/4 cup) plain additive-free
　sheep's milk yoghurt, or plain additive-
　free full-fat Greek-style yoghurt

2 tablespoons nutritional yeast flakes

Preheat the oven to 200°C (400°F/Gas 6) and grease a 28 x 18 x 5 cm (111/4 x 7 x 2 inch) ovenproof dish.

Add 2 tablespoons of the olive oil to a large frying pan over medium heat and gently fry the zucchini for 5–7 minutes, turning frequently, until golden. Remove from the pan and set aside.

Add the remaining olive oil, the onion and garlic to the pan and cook for 5–7 minutes, or until the onion browns. Add the meat and cook for 10 minutes, or until brown. Add the tomatoes, passata, tomato paste and herbs and reduce the heat. Simmer, covered, for 15 minutes and season with salt and pepper to taste.

Add the half the meat mixture to the ovenproof dish, followed by half the zucchini and yoghurt. Repeat and top with the yeast flakes. Bake in the oven, uncovered, for 25 minutes.

Remove from the oven and allow to stand for 10 minutes before serving.

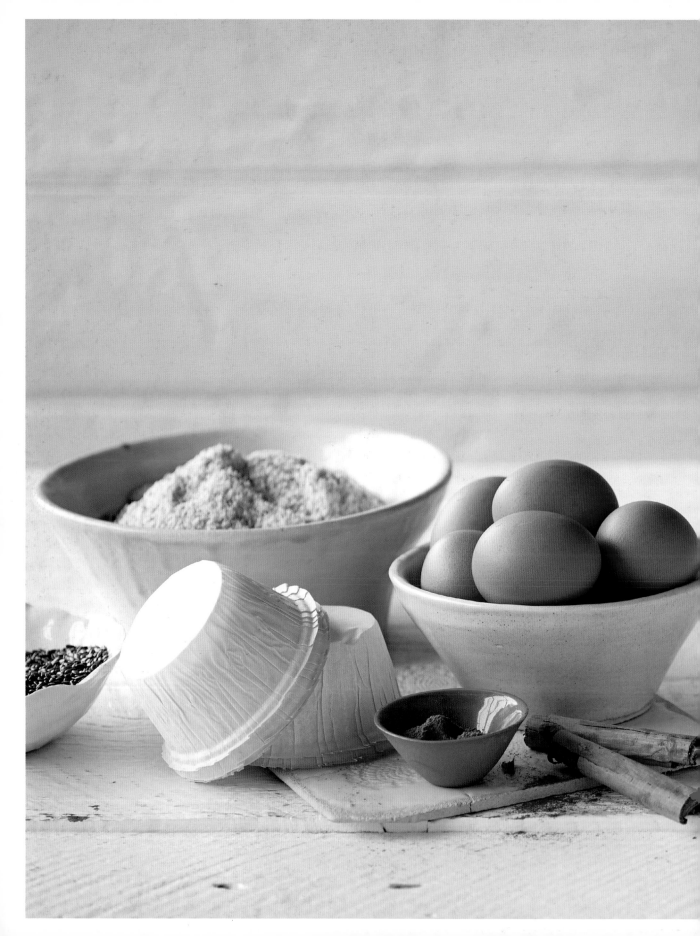

DESSERTS AND BAKING

A great meal requires a matching dessert and ethicurians will be delighted when you bring these show-stopping seasonal desserts to the table. You'll be all about the pudding while eating yourself beautiful in the process. Move over pre-sliced factory bread. Try these no-knead wheat- and yeast-free bread recipes, which have a wonderful texture and flavour. The hearty Chia and Flaxseed loaves, gluten-free crunchy Flat Breads and Oatmeal biscuits will remind you that there's nothing quite like homemade baking.

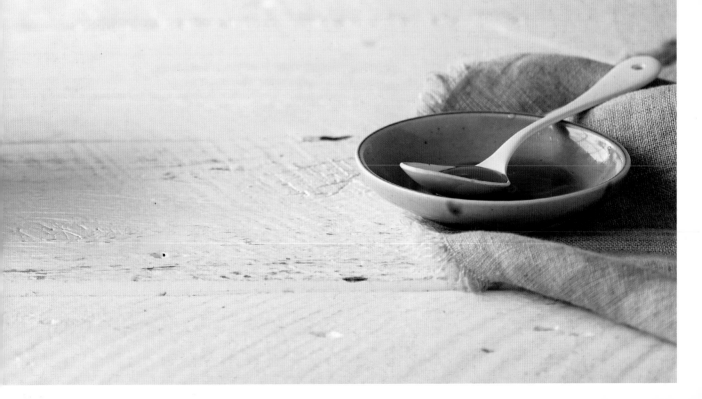

ALMOND MACAROONS

▲WF ▲DF ▲GF ▲SF   MAKES 12

Crunchy on the outside and chewy in the centre, these billowy melt-in-the-mouth macaroons are surprisingly easy to make. Indulge in them while sipping a hot cup of cacao almond milk.

pinch of ground cinnamon

1 teaspoon grated lemon zest

2 organic egg whites

1 teaspoon alcohol-free vanilla extract

2 tablespoons rice malt syrup, or sweetener of your choice

1 teaspoon freshly squeezed lemon juice

125 g (4^{1}/$_{2}$ oz/1^{1}/$_{4}$ cups) coarsely ground almonds

Preheat the oven to 130°C (250°F/Gas 1) and line a baking tray with baking paper.

Place the cinnamon and lemon zest in a medium bowl and mix well.

Using an electric mixer, beat the egg whites and fold into the cinnamon mixture. Add the vanilla, rice malt syrup and lemon juice and stir well to combine. Add the ground almonds and stir again.

Scoop walnut-sized portions of the batter onto the prepared baking tray, and bake on the middle shelf of the oven for 30 minutes.

Remove from the oven and use a spatula to transfer the macaroons to a wire rack to cool.

These are best eaten straight away but will keep in an airtight container for 2–3 days.

▶SUPERCHARGED TIP◀

Save egg yolks by freezing them in ice cube trays until ready for use. Add a pinch of salt to each yolk to stabilise them. They'll last in the freezer for up to 3 months. To use, thaw in the fridge and then mix them well. Leftover egg yolks can also be refrigerated for 3–4 days.

FOOLISH FUDGE BROWNIES

▲WF ▲DF ▲GF ▲SF   MAKES 16

So-named because they are brimming with unusual ingredients that will trick even a health sceptic. Be warned: it is hard to stop at one.

400 g (14 oz) tin black beans,
  rinsed and drained

4 organic eggs

2 tablespoons coconut oil, or 40 g (1¹/₂ oz)
  unsalted butter

2 teaspoons alcohol-free vanilla extract

190 g (6³/₄ oz/1 cup) xylitol

3 tablespoons ground cacao

¹/₂ teaspoon gluten-free baking powder

Celtic sea salt

16 walnut halves

Preheat the oven to 200°C (400°F/Gas 6) and grease and line a 20 x 20 x 4 cm (8 x 8 x 1¹/₂ inch) baking tin.

Using a stick blender or food processor, combine the black beans, eggs, coconut oil, vanilla, xylitol, cacao, baking powder and salt. Process until smooth.

Pour the batter into your prepared baking tin and arrange the walnuts in even rows, 4 across and 4 down.

Bake for 25–30 minutes in the oven or until a skewer inserted in the centre comes out clean.

Cut into 16 squares, ensuring you have a nut piece in the centre of each.

These will keep for a week in an airtight container in the fridge.

▶HEALTH BENEFITS◀

Unlike processed dark chocolate, antioxidants found in raw cacao are preserved in their natural state. These antioxidants have been clinically proven to dissolve plaque that has built up in arteries, helping to reverse heart disease and naturally lower blood pressure.

RASPBERRY-STUDDED PUMPKIN PIE

▲WF ▲DF ▲GF   MAKES 1 PIE

Dig out your pie pans and try this delectable winter warmer. It's a comforting dish bursting with pumpkin, warming spices and hints of vanilla on a crunchy nut base. The raspberries add a sublime luxuriousness with every mouthful.

coconut oil, or unsalted butter, for greasing

BASE

105 g (3¹/₂ oz/²/₃ cup) raw cashew nuts

40 g (1¹/₂ oz/¹/₄ cup) sesame seeds

1¹/₂ tablespoons chia seeds

1¹/₂ tablespoons flaxseeds

40 g (1¹/₂ oz/¹/₄ cup) sunflower seeds

60 g (2¹/₄ oz/¹/₃ cup) cooked brown rice

60 g (2¹/₄ oz/¹/₃ cup) quinoa flakes

6 drops stevia liquid, or 1 tablespoon
   rice malt syrup

1 teaspoon alcohol-free vanilla extract

¹/₂ teaspoon ground cinnamon

2–3 tablespoons coconut oil, or
   40–60 g (1¹/₂–2¹/₄ oz) unsalted butter

TOPPING

600 g (1 lb 5 oz) pumpkin (winter squash)
   or sweet potato, steamed and cooled

1 tablespoon almond milk

2 large organic eggs, beaten

6 drops stevia liquid

1 tablespoon coconut oil

¹/₄ teaspoon ground cinnamon

¹/₄ teaspoon freshly grated nutmeg

1 teaspoon alcohol-free vanilla extract

about 20 raspberries

Preheat the oven to 190°C (375°F/Gas 5) and lightly grease a 20 cm (8 inch) springform cake tin or pie dish.

Combine all the base ingredients in a food processor, adding the coconut oil last, and process for about 15 seconds or until crunchy.

Remove the dough and, using your hands, press it evenly into the prepared tin, packing it slightly around the edges to make a crust. Bake blind for 10–15 minutes or until the base is firm and lightly golden in colour.

To make the topping, combine all the ingredients, except the raspberries, in a large bowl and mash with a fork until smooth.

Spoon the topping over the base and stud with the raspberries. Return the pie to the oven and bake for 35 minutes.

This is delicious served either warm or chilled. It will keep for 5 days in an airtight container in the fridge.

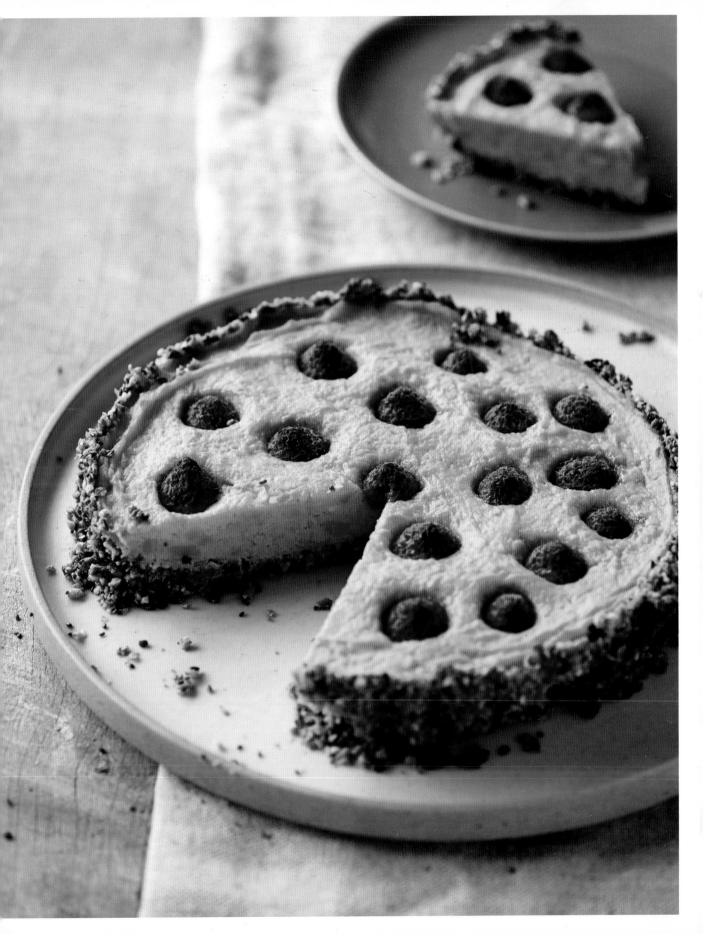

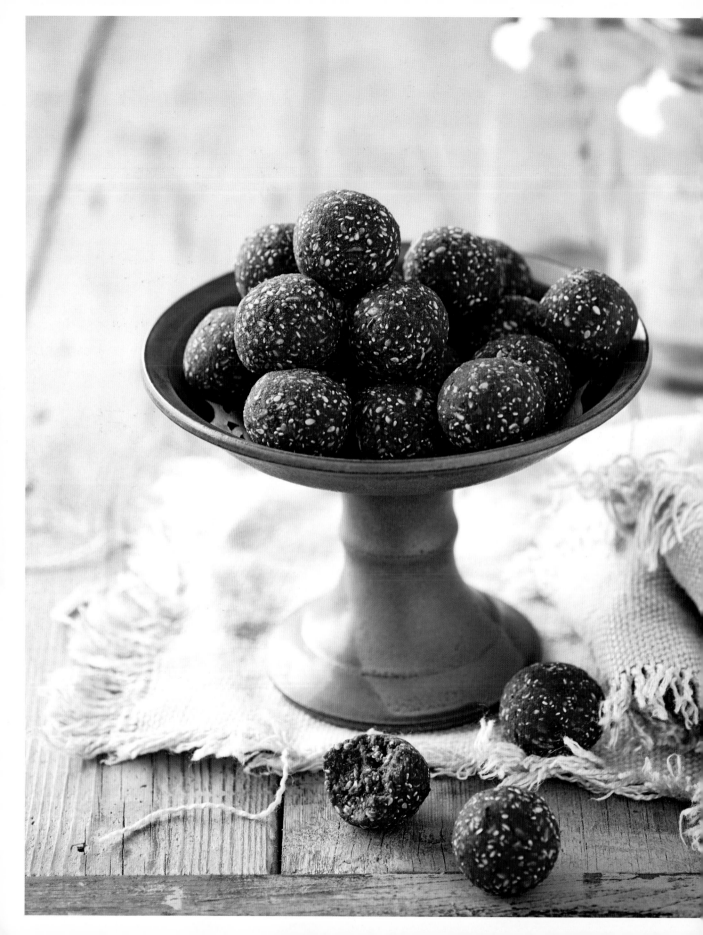

CHOCOLATE TRUFFLES

▲WF ▲DF ▲GF ▲SF ▲VG   MAKES 28 TRUFFLES

These are not exactly textbook truffles, but take a walk over to the dark side and you'll discover that they are they are delicious, texturally-sound and will fit the bill when you're in need of a chocolate fix.

250 ml (9 fl oz/1 cup) additive-free
  coconut milk

125 g (4¹/2 oz) nut butter

30 g (1 oz/¹/4 cup) ground cacao

60 g (2¹/4 oz/¹/2 cup) chia seeds

75 g (2¹/2 oz/¹/2 cup) sesame seeds

75 g (2¹/2 oz/¹/2 cup) pepitas
  (pumpkin seeds)

75 g (2¹/2 oz/¹/2 cup) sunflower seeds

75 g (2¹/2 oz/¹/2 cup) coconut flour

2¹/2 tablespoons rice malt syrup,
  or sweetener of your choice

Place all the ingredients in a food processor and pulse until smooth.

Remove 1 tablespoon of the mixture and use your hands to form a small ball. Repeat with the remaining mixture until you have used it all.

These will keep in an airtight container in the fridge for 2 weeks, and in the freezer for 3 months.

▶SUPERCHARGED TIP◀

Blending chia seeds makes them more bio-available for the body. These truffles are also delicious rolled in grated coconut.

BLUEBERRY AND COCONUT MUFFINS

▲WF ▲GF   MAKES 12

*Steer clear of the huge cakes that have invaded our supermarket shelves, they're usually full
of additives and sugar. Remember the golden rule: the best muffin is the one you bake yourself.*

250 ml (9 fl oz/1 cup) almond or rice milk

30 g (1 oz/1/4 cup) chia seeds

130 g (41/2 oz/1 cup) coconut flour

1/2 teaspoon bicarbonate of soda
   (baking soda)

1/2 teaspoon gluten-free baking powder

1/4 teaspoon sea salt

1 teaspoon alcohol-free vanilla extract

140 g (5 oz/1 cup) coconut palm sugar

5 organic eggs

125 g (41/2 oz) unsalted butter, melted

155 g (51/2 oz/1 cup) fresh blueberries
   (see note)

Preheat the oven to 175°C (345°F/Gas 3–4) and place paper
liners in a 6-hole (80 ml/21/2 fl oz/1/3 cup) muffin tin.

Mix 125 ml (4 fl oz/1/2 cup) of the milk with the chia seeds.
Set aside for 30 minutes.

In a bowl, mix the coconut flour, bicarbonate of soda, baking
powder, salt, vanilla and coconut palm sugar together.

In a separate bowl, mix the eggs, butter and remaining
milk and stir in the blueberries, flour mixture and chia
seed mixture.

Divide the mixture among the prepared muffin holes
and bake for 40 minutes, or until a skewer inserted into a
muffin comes out clean.

These will keep in the fridge in an airtight container
for 5 days, or out of the fridge in an airtight container
for 2 days.

NOTE: If fresh blueberries aren't in season, use 125 g
(41/2 oz/1 cup) frozen berries instead.

▶SUPERCHARGED TIP◀

You can mix it up by changing the fruit you toss in this mix.
Fresh bananas or raspberries work well too.

CHIA SEED STARS

▲WF ▲DF ▲GF ▲SF   MAKES 12

If you fancy a rainy day baking session, roll out these star-studded biscuits. Packed with countless micronutrients important for DNA replication and the breakdown of carbohydrate into energy, these are perfect for when people turn up for afternoon tea.

95–145 g (3¼–5¼ oz) gluten-free
  rolled oats

50 g (1¾ oz/½ cup) almond meal

1 teaspoon gluten-free baking powder

1 tablespoon chia seeds

2 tablespoons shredded coconut

2 organic eggs

70 g (2½ oz) coconut butter

1 tablespoon rice malt syrup, or 6 drops
  stevia liquid

180 g (6¼ oz) almond butter

1 teaspoon alcohol-free vanilla extract

Preheat the oven to 175°C (345°F/Gas 3–4) and line a baking tray with baking paper.

Mix the oats, almond meal, baking powder, chia seeds and shredded coconut together in a medium bowl.

In a separate bowl, whisk the eggs and add the coconut butter, rice malt syrup or stevia, almond butter and vanilla and stir until combined. Stir through the oat mixture and let the dough sit for a few minutes – this will make it easier to work with.

Lightly dust a clean work surface with gluten-free flour. Using your hands, work the dough into a ball. Roll it out onto the floured work surface and use a star cutter to cut out the shapes.

Place on the baking tray and cook in the oven for 12 minutes. Turn out onto a wire rack to cool.

The chia seed stars will keep for 1 week in an airtight container.

LAYERED QUINOA TRIFLE

▲WF ▲GF   SERVES 4

Layers and layers of health-promoting ingredients make this Christmassy dessert one you can indulge in all year round.

100 g (3¹/2 oz/¹/2 cup) quinoa

¹/2 teaspoon ground cinnamon

pinch of Celtic sea salt

60 ml (2 fl oz/¹/4 cup) unsweetened almond milk

¹/2 teaspoon alcohol-free vanilla extract

6 drops stevia liquid, or 1 tablespoon rice malt syrup

1 tablespoon slivered almonds

2 bananas, sliced

130 g (4³/4 oz/¹/2 cup) full-fat Greek-style yoghurt

4 tablespoons coconut flakes

110 g (3³/4 oz/¹/2 cup) mixed berries

1 teaspoon almond butter, melted

1 tablespoon chia seeds, for sprinkling

Place the quinoa in a fine-mesh sieve. Rinse with cold running water for 2–3 minutes, moving the seeds around with your hand to ensure that the seeds are well rinsed and any residue is removed. Bring 250 ml (9 fl oz/1 cup) water to the boil in a large saucepan. Add the quinoa, return to the boil, cover and reduce the heat to low for 12–15 minutes or until all the water has been absorbed. Remove from the heat and set aside to cool.

Place the quinoa in a bowl and stir through the cinnamon and salt.

In a saucepan over medium–low heat, warm the almond milk for 3–4 minutes. Stir in the vanilla and stevia or rice malt syrup.

Add a couple of spoons of quinoa to four glass jars, or glasses. Mix through the almond milk and follow with layers of slivered almonds, banana slices, yoghurt, coconut flakes and berries. Repeat until the jars are full, with berries as the top layer.

Top with the melted almond butter and chia seeds.

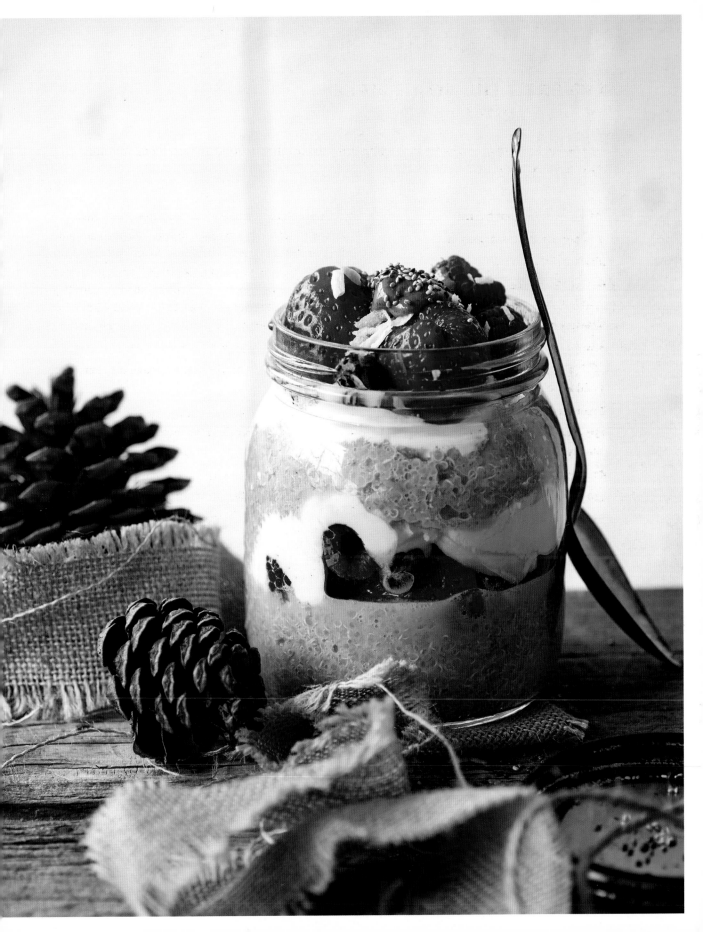

BROWN RICE PUDDING

▲WF ▲DF ▲GF ▲VG   SERVES 2–3

The sweetness of the blueberries mingles with the nuttiness of the brown rice to create this deliciously fragrant rice pudding, both rich in antioxidants and delightfully low in sugar. This is the definitive little pudding that could.

370 g (12³⁄₄ oz/2 cups) cooked brown rice

375 ml (13 fl oz/1¹⁄₂ cups) almond milk

125 ml (4 fl oz/¹⁄₂ cup) additive-free
  coconut milk

1 teaspoon stevia powder

juice of ¹⁄₂ lemon

1 teaspoon grated lemon zest

1 teaspoon ground cinnamon

¹⁄₄ teaspoon ground cardamom

pinch of freshly grated nutmeg

155 g (5¹⁄₂ oz/1 cup) fresh blueberries

ground cinnamon, to serve

Put the rice, almond milk, coconut milk, stevia, lemon juice and zest, cinnamon, cardamom and nutmeg in a saucepan and cook over medium heat, stirring often, for about 10 minutes, or until it starts to thicken and become creamy. Reduce the heat to low, add the blueberries, and stir for a few more minutes.

Spoon into serving bowls and sprinkle generously with cinnamon.

NOTE: You can also add 20 g (³⁄₄ oz) of unsalted butter when you add the almond milk if it takes your fancy, but it will no longer be dairy-free.

VERY BERRY CHEESECAKE

▲WF ▲DF ▲GF ▲VG   MAKES 1

In addition to Vitamin E and iron, this supercharged Very Berry Cheesecake is a rich source of phytonutrients. Berries are one of the highest sources of plant-based chemical resveratrol, a powerful anti-inflammatory.

BASE

120 g (4¼ oz/¾ cup) raw cashew nuts

55 g (2 oz/¾ cup) additive-free
  shredded coconut

¼ teaspoon stevia powder

60 ml (2 fl oz/¼ cup) freshly squeezed
  lemon juice

20 g (¾ oz) coconut butter, melted

FILLING

310 g (11 oz/2 cups) raw cashew nuts

70 g (2½ oz) coconut butter

125 g (4½ oz/1 cup) mixed frozen berries

1 teaspoon alcohol-free vanilla extract

1 tablespoon freshly squeezed lemon juice

¼ teaspoon stevia powder

80 ml (2½ fl oz/⅓ cup) additive-free
  coconut milk

75 g (2¾ oz/½ cup) fresh berries,
  for decorating

To make the base, process the nuts and coconut in a blender until finely chopped.

Stir in the remaining ingredients, adding some filtered water if necessary – the mixture should be stiff and hold together while not being too crumbly.

Using your hands, mould into a dough and press into a 16 cm (6¼ inch) springform cake tin. Place in the freezer for 20 minutes.

To make the filling, process all the ingredients, except the fresh berries, in a blender until smooth.

Remove the base from the freezer and smooth the filling over it with a spatula.

Return the cake tin to the freezer, or fridge, for about 20–30 minutes, or until set.

Top with fresh berries to serve.

BERRIES WITH ACV AND CASHEW NUT CREAM

▲WF ▲DF ▲GF ▲VG   SERVES 2

This dessert is very definitely worth a try. It may look simple and understated but the addition of apple cider vinegar (ACV) will ensure you never eat berries on their own again. This is the perfect end to a dinner party.

440 g (15¹/₂ oz/2 cups) fresh berries

2 teaspoons apple cider vinegar

45 g (1¹/₂ oz/¹/₃ cup) slivered almonds

CASHEW NUT CREAM
155 g (5¹/₂ oz/1 cup) raw cashew nuts
   (see note)

170 ml (5¹/₂ fl oz/²/₃ cup) filtered water

8 drops stevia liquid

1 teaspoon alcohol-free vanilla
   extract (optional)

To make the cashew nut cream, place all the ingredients in a food processor and whizz until smooth and creamy. Add a little water if the mixture isn't smooth.

Divide the berries between two small bowls. Pour the vinegar evenly over each, top with slivered almonds and the cashew nut cream, and serve.

NOTE: The cashew nut cream can be stored in the fridge in a covered container for up to 1 week. You can substitute the same quantity of almonds, sunflower seeds, macadamias or hazelnuts for the cashews.

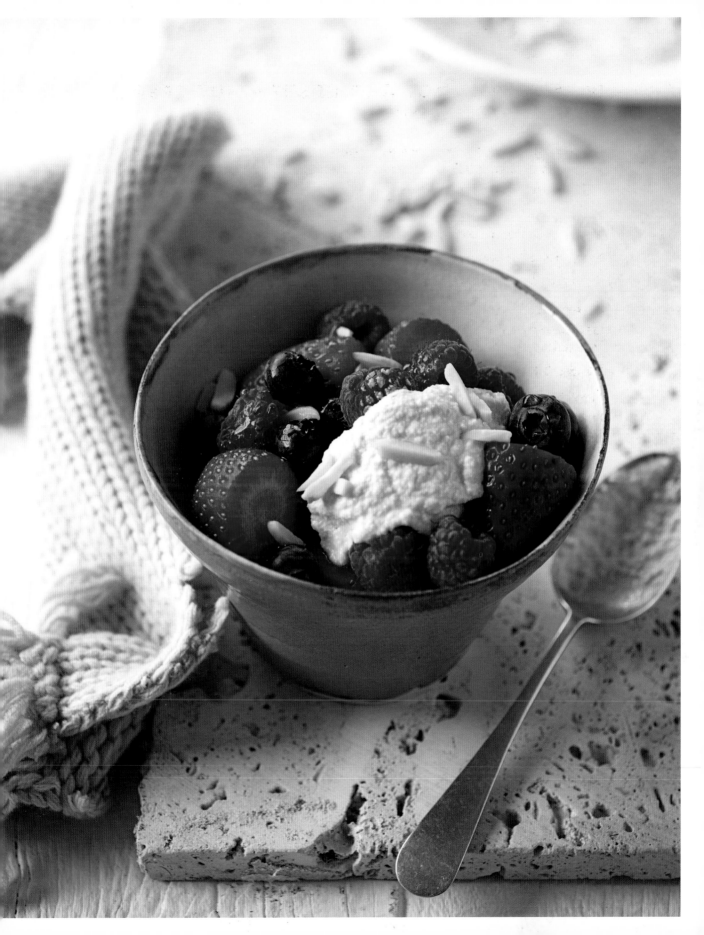

AVOCADO AND CHOCOLATE MOUSSE

▲WF ▲DF ▲GF ▲SF ▲VG   SERVES 2

Avocado is a supercharged food which boasts an impressive résumé. Full of monounsaturated good fats it not only helps boost your good (HDL) cholesterol, but can help lower your bad (LDL) cholesterol too. All of these luscious good fats have another beneficial effect: they help your skin and locks glow. Hooray for chocolate mousse!

1 ripe avocado, peeled and stone removed

60 ml (2 fl oz/¼ cup) almond milk

1 tablespoon chia seeds

1 teaspoon alcohol-free vanilla extract

4 tablespoons ground cacao

8 drops stevia liquid, or sweetener of your choice

Combine all the ingredients in a blender and blend for 30 seconds, or until smooth and creamy.

Spoon the mousse into two glass jars or cups and chill slightly before serving.

HEALTHY CARROT CAKE

▲WF ▲GF ▲SF   MAKES 1 CAKE

This scrummy carrot cake really lives up to its name, containing no gluten and no sugar. In fact, you can rest assured that with every bite you are bringing health and vitality into your body. It embodies everything that a carrot cake should be, along with a luscious creamy icing.

150 g (5^1/2 oz/1^1/2 cups) almond meal, or gluten-free flour of your choice

60 g (2^1/4 oz/^{1}/2 cup) chopped walnuts

^{1}/2 teaspoon gluten-free baking powder

1 teaspoon bicarbonate of soda (baking soda)

^{1}/4 teaspoon sea salt

1 teaspoon ground cinnamon

^{1}/2 teaspoon freshly grated nutmeg

^{3}/4 teaspoon stevia powder

2 organic eggs, beaten

60 g (2^1/4 oz) unsalted butter, melted

80 ml (2^1/2 fl oz/^{1}/3 cup) additive-free coconut milk

200 g (7 oz) grated carrot

CREAMY CASHEW COCONUT ICING

120 g (4^1/4 oz/^{3}/4 cup) raw cashew nuts

400 g (14 oz) tin coconut cream

finely grated zest of 1 lemon

juice of 1 lemon

5–6 drops stevia liquid

Preheat the oven to 170°C (325°F/Gas 3) and grease an 18 cm (7 inch) round cake tin.

Place the almond flour, walnuts, baking powder, bicarbonate of soda, salt, cinnamon, nutmeg and stevia in a bowl and stir to combine.

In a separate bowl, whisk the eggs, butter and coconut milk together. Add to the dry ingredients and fold through.

Squeeze the excess water out of the carrot (using your hands is best) then add the carrot to the bowl. Fold in lightly.

Spoon the mixture into the prepared tin and bake for 45 minutes, or until the cake springs back when pressed in the centre.

Turn out onto a wire rack to cool.

To make the icing, place the cashews, half the coconut cream, the lemon zest and juice in a food processor and blitz for a few minutes, slowly adding more coconut cream until it reaches a smooth consistency. Add the stevia, blitzing little by little, until you get the desired sweetness of your icing. Place in the coldest section of your fridge to thicken while the cake cools. (You could also put it in the freezer for 5–10 minutes to speed up the thickening.)

When the cake has cooled, spoon your icing all over the top. This cake will keep for 5 days in an airtight container.

▶**HEALTH BENEFITS**◀

Carrots contain Vitamins B, C, D, E and K and beta-carotene, and the minerals calcium, iron, phosphorus, chromium, magnesium, potassium and silica. Carrots are excellent for skin problems, and have been known to have great healing effects on ulcerous and inflamed conditions of the stomach and intestines.

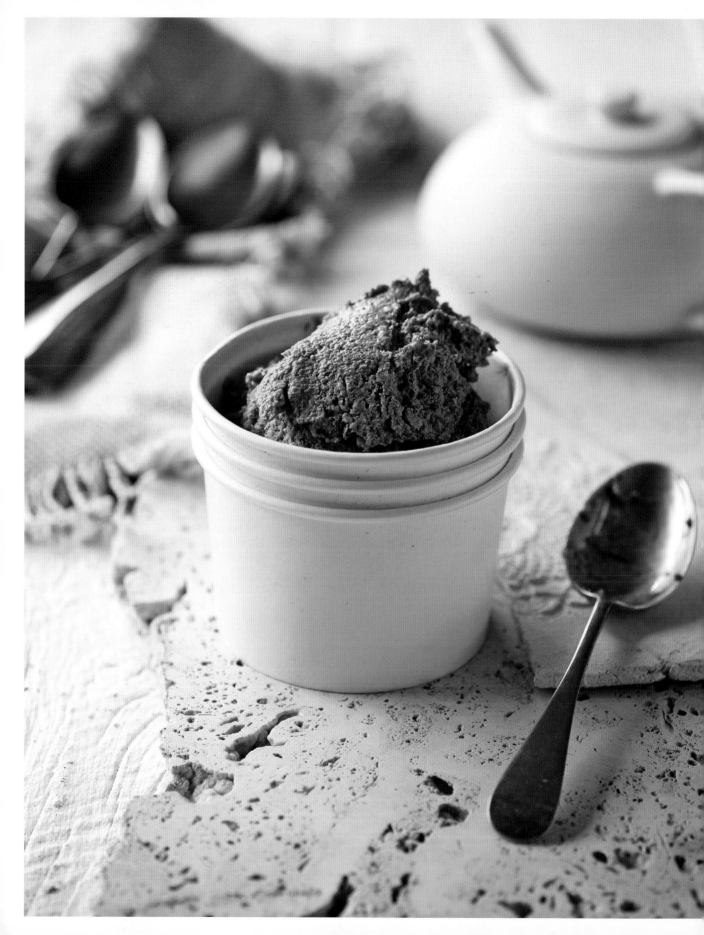

RASPBERRY GELATO

▲WF ▲DF ▲GF ▲VG   SERVES 3

A low-maintenance gelato that will sweep you away with its astonishing taste and deliver maximum refreshment on sunny days.

195 g (6³/4 oz/1¹/4 cups) raw cashew nuts

2 teaspoons alcohol-free vanilla extract

105 g (3¹/2 oz/³/4 cup) frozen raspberries

1 tablespoon freshly squeezed lemon juice

6 drops stevia liquid

125 ml (4 fl oz/¹/2 cup) additive-free coconut milk

Place all the ingredients in a high speed food processor and blend until smooth. Transfer into three individual ice cream moulds or ramekins.

Place in the freezer for 2 hours, or until they have set.

Remove from the moulds before serving by running a warm knife along the inside edge of the moulds.

▶HEALTH BENEFITS◀

Raspberries are an exceptional food that are rich in antioxidants that help reduce the visible signs of aging.

HOME-STYLE APPLE CRUMBLE

▲WF ▲GF   SERVES 2

Traditional homemade apple crumble is one of my favourite desserts. This one is layered with juicy apples and a crunchy nut topping.

4–5 granny smith apples, washed, cored and sliced

1/2 teaspoon freshly grated nutmeg

1/4 teaspoon stevia powder

1/2 teaspoon ground cinnamon

175 g (6 oz/1 1/2 cups) walnuts (see note)

60 g (2 1/4 oz) unsalted butter, cut into cubes, plus extra for greasing

pinch of Celtic sea salt

Preheat the oven to 175°C (345°F/Gas 3–4) and grease a square 20 x 20 cm (8 x 8 inch) ovenproof dish.

Place the apple slices in a bowl with the nutmeg, stevia and cinnamon and toss so the apples are evenly coated in the spice mix.

Place the apple slices in a layer in the prepared dish.

In a food processor, process the nuts until fine. Add the butter and salt and blitz until crumbly.

Sprinkle the nut mixture over the apples and cook in the oven for 25 minutes, or until crispy on top.

NOTE: If you don't like walnuts, substitute with the same quantity of almonds or mixed nuts.

▶HEALTH BENEFITS◀

If you are on an intense sugar-free diet, you will need to eliminate all fruit from your diet which will also eliminate the proliferation of pathogenic yeast. However, once the gut has healed, selected fruits, if combined with other easily digested foods, are a suitable low-sugar snack for when cravings strike. The fructose-to-fibre content in tart and tangy granny smith apples is not extreme, and therefore easier for your gut to break down and digest. They're a fantastic choice if you're looking for a fruity dessert but don't want to indulge in high-sugar fruits.

EASY SWEET POTATO ICE CREAM

▲WF ▲DF ▲GF ▲SF ▲VG   SERVES 2

If you've never tasted sweet potato ice cream you are in for an unexpected treat. I can guarantee that this recipe will soon become one of your favourite beautifying desserts and turn you into an underground flavour hunter.

150 g (5¹/₂ oz) sweet potato, cooked
  and puréed

400 ml (14 fl oz) additive-free coconut milk

1 tablespoon ground cacao

6 drops stevia liquid, or sweetener
  of your choice

20 g (³/₄ oz) almond butter

Place all the ingredients in a food processor and purée until well blended, scraping down the sides with a spatula as required. Transfer to a freezer-proof dish and freeze for 20 minutes.

This ice cream will keep in the freezer for 2 weeks.

▶SUPERCHARGED TIP◀

This ice cream is best eaten immediately after you remove it from the freezer. It also has a tendency to become icier the longer it's in the freezer.

OATMEAL BISCUITS

▲WF ▲GF   MAKES 10–12

You'll be taken aback by the simplicity of these all-star fibre-rich biscuits, which contain ingredients that not only soak up cholesterol but also help to smooth out wrinkles.

145 g (5¼ oz) gluten-free rolled oats

35 g (1¼ oz/¼ cup) coconut flour

25 g (1 oz/¼ cup) almond meal

½ teaspoon ground cinnamon

½ teaspoon freshly grated nutmeg

1 teaspoon stevia powder

½ teaspoon sea salt

1 organic egg, whisked

⅓ cup unsweetened apple sauce
  or mashed banana

60 g (2¼ oz) unsalted butter, melted

1 teaspoon alcohol-free vanilla extract

Preheat the oven to 190°C (375°F/Gas 5) and line a baking tray with baking paper.

Place the oats, coconut flour, almond meal, cinnamon, nutmeg, stevia and salt in a bowl and stir to combine.

Place all the remaining ingredients in a small bowl and whisk together.

Add the wet ingredients to the dry and mix with a wooden spoon until combined.

Scoop out handfuls of dough, roll them into balls and place them on the prepared baking tray, pressing down with a spatula until they are about 5 cm (2 inches) wide and 1–2 cm (½–¾ inch) thick.

Bake in the oven for 12 minutes, or until they are golden.

Remove from the oven and transfer to a wire rack to cool.

These biscuits will keep for 2 weeks in an airtight container.

⟫ **SUPERCHARGED TIP** ⟪

To make apple sauce, just peel, core and cut up 3–4 green apples into 2.5 cm (1 inch) chunks. Place them in a saucepan and add 2 teaspoons of lemon juice. Stir, then add enough water to cover them and a pinch of ground cinnamon, freshly grated nutmeg and Celtic sea salt. Bring to a boil then simmer for 20–30 minutes, or until soft and mushy. Use a masher to remove any lumps.

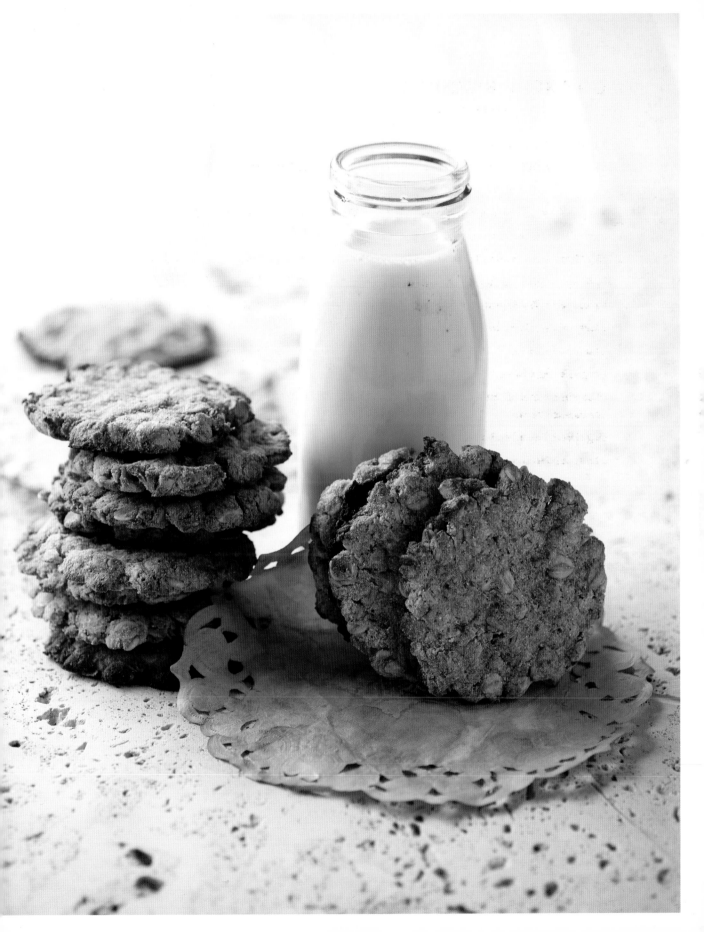

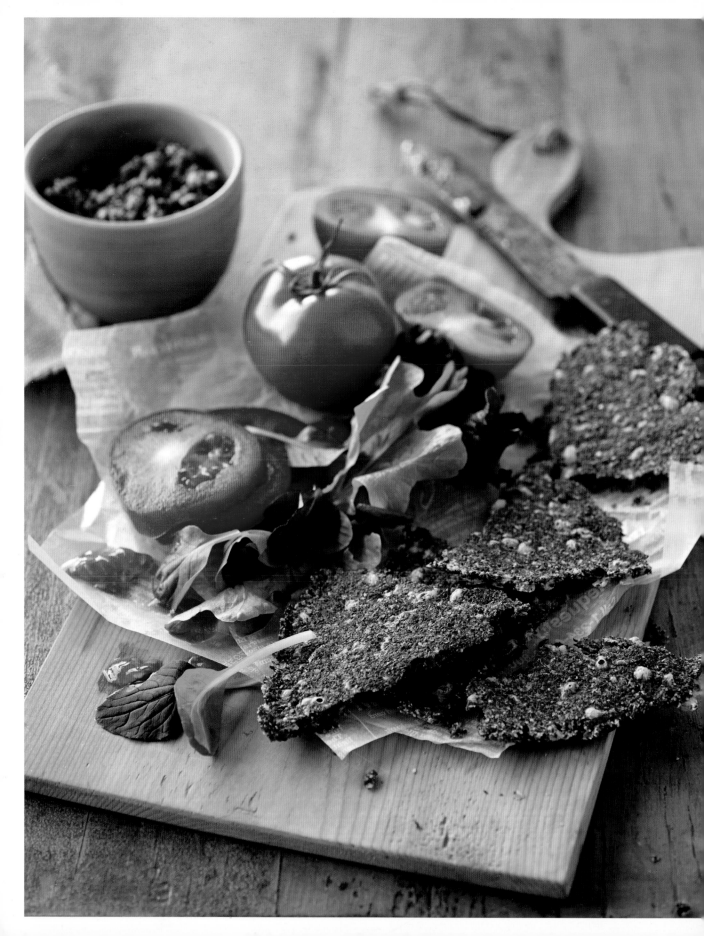

SNAPPY FLAX CRACKERS

▲WF ▲GF ▲SF ▲VG   MAKES 12–14

Holy smoke, these are good. If you're looking for a quick and easy way to make crackers but don't want to go to too much effort these are for you. With only four ingredients they're a snap to make and are delicious topped with pâté, dip, avocado spread or anything else you might be hankering for.

100 g (3¹/₂ oz/1 cup) flaxseed meal

30 g (1 oz/¹/₃ cup) coarsely grated parmesan cheese

¹/₂ teaspoon sea salt

125 ml (4 fl oz/¹/₂ cup) filtered water

Preheat the oven to 200°C (400°F/Gas 6).

Mix all the ingredients together in a bowl.

Spoon the mixture onto a baking tray, pressing it down firmly so the mixture is about 3 mm (¹/₈ inch) thick.

Cook in the oven for 15 minutes, then transfer on the tray to a wire rack to cool down and crisp up.

Once crispy, use a spatula to carefully lift the cracker away from the tray. Break into bite-sized pieces.

The crackers will keep in an airtight container for 2–3 weeks.

▶HEALTH BENEFITS◀

Flaxseed is one of the most concentrated plant sources of omega-3s. Flaxseed and linseeds are the same thing.

SPINACH LOAF

▲WF ▲GF ▲SF   MAKES 1 LOAF

The best way to eat bread worthy of a beautiful you is to make it yourself. Enter an elegant combination of two of my existing recipes, spinach toast and zucchini loaf. I love both recipes but wanted to unite the health benefits of spinach toast into the texture and generous height of a traditional loaf. It's the perfect loaf for mopping up soup and feeding a crowd.

250 g (9 oz/2¹/₂ cups) almond flour

¹/₄ teaspoon Celtic sea salt

1¹/₂ teaspoons gluten-free baking powder

¹/₄ teaspoon bicarbonate of soda
(baking soda)

2 bunches English spinach, stems removed,
leaves blanched and drained

3 organic eggs, beaten

60 ml (2 fl oz/¹/₄ cup) additive-free
coconut milk

1 teaspoon freshly squeezed lemon juice

60 g (2¹/₄ oz) unsalted butter, melted

1 tablespoon apple cider vinegar

Preheat the oven to 175°C (345°F/Gas 3–4) and grease and line a 20 x 9 cm (8 x 3¹/₂ inch) loaf (bar) tin with baking paper.

In a large bowl, combine the almond flour, salt, baking powder and bicarbonate of soda.

Whizz the spinach leaves in a food processor (or chop them finely) and add to the bowl, along with the eggs, coconut milk, lemon juice, butter and vinegar. Mix thoroughly.

Spoon the mixture into the prepared tin and level the surface with the back of a spoon dipped in cold water.

Bake the loaf on the middle rack of the oven for about 45 minutes, or until a skewer inserted in the centre comes out clean.

Turn out onto a wire rack to cool, then enjoy!

This loaf will keep for up to 1 week in an airtight container in the fridge, or can be frozen for up to 1 month.

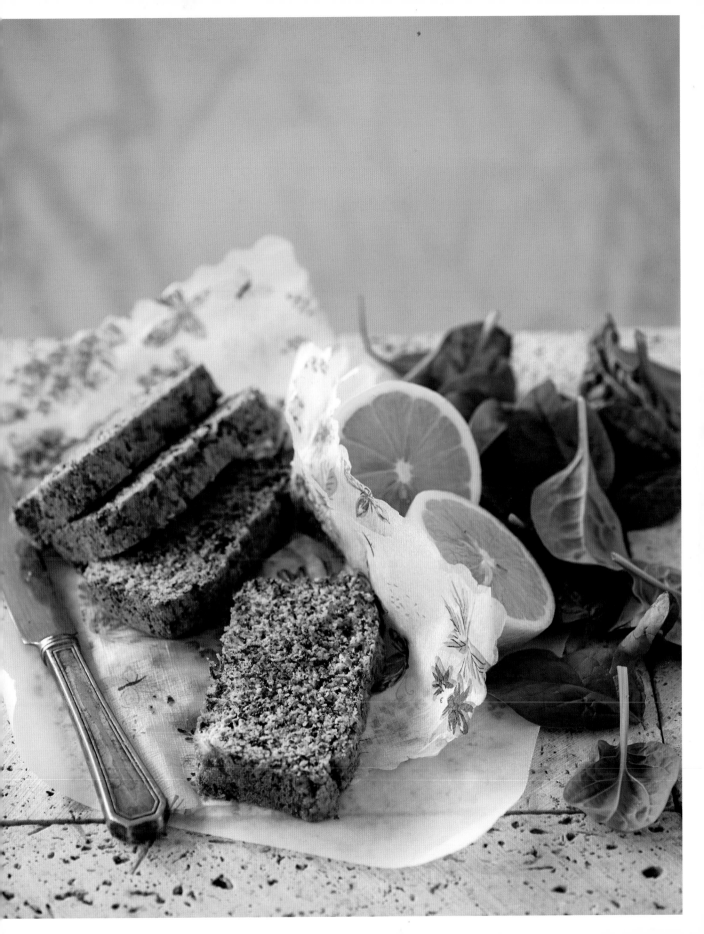

GLUTEN-FREE LOAF

▲WF ▲DF ▲GF ▲SF ▲VG   MAKES 1 LOAF

Packed full of good fats, this everyday gluten-free loaf is naturally rich in antioxidants that your body will enjoy. When it comes to satisfaction, this loaf is off the scale and is a natural companion to delicious dips in any picnic hamper.

150 g (5¹/₂ oz/1¹/₂ cups) almond meal

95 g (3¹/₄ oz/³/₄ cup) ground arrowroot

30 g (1 oz/¹/₄ cup) golden flaxmeal

¹/₂ teaspoon stevia powder

pinch of Celtic sea salt

¹/₂ teaspoon gluten-free baking powder

1 teaspoon bicarbonate of soda
  (baking soda)

4 organic eggs

1 teaspoon rice malt syrup

1 teaspoon apple cider vinegar

Preheat the oven to 175°C (345°F/Gas 3–4) and grease and line a 20 x 10 x 6 cm (8 x 4 x 2¹/₂ inch) loaf (bar) tin with baking paper.

Combine the almond meal, arrowroot, flaxmeal, stevia, salt, baking powder and bicarbonate of soda in a large bowl.

In a separate bowl, whisk the eggs until they are light and fluffy. Add the rice malt syrup and vinegar and stir well to combine.

Transfer the wet ingredients into the almond meal mixture and use a wooden spoon to combine.

Spoon the mixture into the prepared tin and bake in the oven for 30–35 minutes, or until a skewer inserted in the centre comes out clean.

Remove from the oven and transfer to a wire rack to cool.

This bread will keep in the fridge for 1 week and the freezer for 2 months.

▶ HEALTH BENEFITS ◀

Golden flaxmeal is the product left after pressing flaxseeds to get flaxseed oil. It still contains 12% fat, half of this fat being the omega-3 essential fatty acid, alpha-linolenic acid (ALA).

CRUNCHY FLAT BREAD

▲WF ▲DF ▲GF ▲SF   MAKES 2 FLAT BREADS

This is so quick to make (just 12 minutes in the oven) and so satisfying. And versatile – you can add whatever toppings you like or break it up and use as a vehicle for dips.

150 g (5¹/2 oz/1¹/2 cups) almond meal

¹/4 teaspoon Celtic sea salt

¹/4 teaspoon gluten-free baking powder

1 tablespoon extra virgin olive oil

1 organic egg, whisked

1 tablespoon apple cider vinegar

Preheat the oven to 175°C (345°F/Gas 3–4).

Combine the almond meal, salt and baking powder in a large bowl. Add the olive oil, using your fingertips to rub it into the mixture to form a crumble. Add the egg and vinegar and, using a wooden spoon, stir to combine.

Using your hands, take the mixture out of the bowl and transfer to a clean work surface. Roll it into a ball – it will feel quite sticky but knead it for a few minutes until a smooth dough forms. Divide it into two and let it sit on the work surface for 5–10 minutes.

Cut out four pieces of baking paper, approximately 20 x 20 cm (8 x 8 inches), and lay one piece out on the work surface. Transfer a piece of the dough onto the baking paper and add another piece of baking paper to the top. Using a rolling pin, roll out the dough to form a circle about 15 cm (6 inches) in diameter and about 1 cm (¹/2 inch) thick. Repeat with the other ball of dough.

Gently peel off the top layer of baking paper and lift the dough and the bottom layer of baking paper onto a baking tray. Transfer to the oven and bake for 12 minutes, or until golden.

Remove from the oven and peel off the baking paper – it should come away quite easily. Transfer to a wire rack to cool until it's crunchy.

▶SUPERCHARGED TIP◀

Apple cider vinegar is a useful ingredient and one I turn to more and more these days. With a myriad of applications, it can serve as an ever-ready topical astringent for troubled skin, and will draw out toxins from your body when added to a warm bath. Pour 125 ml (4 fl oz/¹/2 cup) of apple cider vinegar and sprinkle ¹/2 cup of Epsom salts into a warm running bath, hop in and relax. This will help to relieve joint pain too.

SWEET POTATO BREAD

▲WF ▲GF ▲SF   MAKES 1 LOAF

Potato flour? Meh. I don't think so. Mash up the real thing and benefit from the Vitamin C to accelerate wound healing, produce collagen – which helps maintain skin's youthful elasticity – and keep your stress levels down.

375 g (13 oz/1½ cups) cooked and mashed sweet potato

1 teaspoon alcohol-free vanilla extract

1 tablespoon apple cider vinegar

1 teaspoon ground ginger

1 teaspoon cinnamon

1 tablespoon rice malt syrup, or sweetener of your choice

60 g (2¼ oz) unsalted butter

3 organic eggs

200 g (7 oz/2 cups) almond meal

1 teaspoon Celtic sea salt

1 teaspoon bicarbonate of soda (baking soda)

Preheat the oven to 175°C (345°F/Gas 3–4) and grease and line a 20 x 9 cm (8 x 3½ inch) loaf (bar) tin with baking paper.

Place the sweet potato, vanilla, vinegar, spices, rice malt syrup and butter in a bowl and stir to combine.

In a separate bowl, use an electric beater to whisk the eggs. Add to the sweet potato mixture with the remaining ingredients.

Spoon into the prepared tin and bake in the oven for 50 minutes, or until a skewer inserted in the centre of the loaf comes out clean.

Turn out onto a wire rack to cool.

COCONUT WRAP

▲WF ▲GF ▲SF   MAKES 2 WRAPS

Encase sandwich fillings or the delicious Chicken and Homemade Mayo Salad (see page 142) with this wrap, or lay it flat and drop on toppings of choice. Goat's cheese and rocket complement it well.

2 organic egg whites, whisked

2 tablespoons coconut flour

1/8 teaspoon bicarbonate of soda (baking soda)

1/8 teaspoon gluten-free baking powder

pinch of Celtic sea salt

60 ml (2 fl oz/1/4 cup) almond milk

20 g (3/4 oz) unsalted butter

Combine all the ingredients except the butter in a large bowl and stir well, ensuring all lumps are removed.

Heat the butter in a large heavy-based frying pan over medium heat. Pour in half the mixture, spreading it over the entire base of the pan.

Cook for 5–7 minutes, or until the mixture starts to bubble. Using a spatula, carefully flip over the mixture and cook on the other side for 5–7 minutes.

Remove from the pan and repeat with the remaining mixture. Cool before serving with your favourite toppings.

NOTE: You can also use this mixture to make 4 flatbreads – simply follow the instructions above, using a quarter of the mixture at a time rather than half.

CHIA AND FLAXSEED LOAF

▲WF ▲GF ▲SF   MAKES 1 LOAF

This is my daily bread and what a diva of a loaf it is. Use it for blissful open-top sandwiches or a mouthwatering and satisfying toasted sandwich. The perfect skin food.

350 g (12 oz/2¹/₃ cups) gluten-free
  self-raising flour

30 g (1 oz/¹/₄ cup) ground flaxseeds

20 g (³/₄ oz/¹/₄ cup) chia seeds

115 g (4 oz/³/₄ cup) mixed sunflower
  seeds and pepitas (pumpkin seeds)

¹/₂ teaspoon sea salt

4 organic eggs

1 teaspoon apple cider vinegar

80 g (2³/₄ oz) unsalted butter, melted

80 ml (2¹/₂ fl oz/¹/₃ cup) additive-free
  coconut milk

6 drops stevia liquid

125 ml (4 fl oz/¹/₂ cup) filtered water

Preheat the oven to 175°C (345°F/Gas 3–4) and grease and line a 20 x 9 cm (8 x 3¹/₂ inch) loaf (bar) tin with baking paper.

Combine the flour, ground flaxseeds, chia and sunflower seeds, pepitas and salt in a bowl and mix until combined.

In a separate large bowl, use an electric beater to beat the eggs for about 2 minutes – they should be pale and fluffy. Stir in the vinegar, butter, coconut milk, stevia and water. Pour the wet ingredients into the bowl with the flour mixture and stir well to combine.

Spoon the mixture into the prepared loaf tin and bake in the oven for 40 minutes, or until a skewer inserted in the centre of the loaf comes out clean.

Turn out onto a wire rack to cool.

This loaf will keep for 1 week in the fridge or 2 months in the freezer.

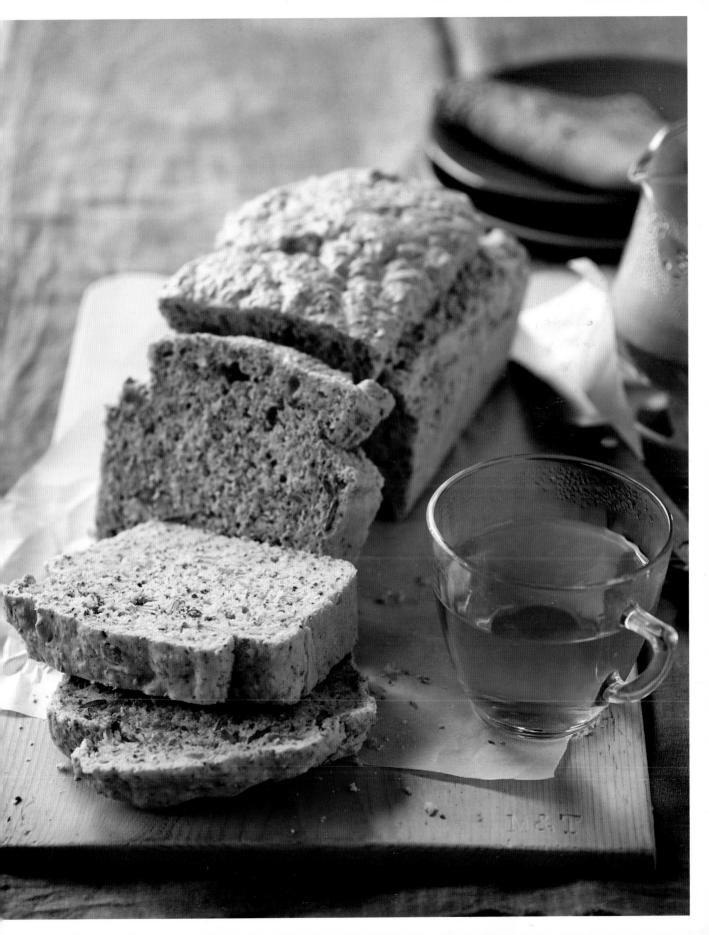

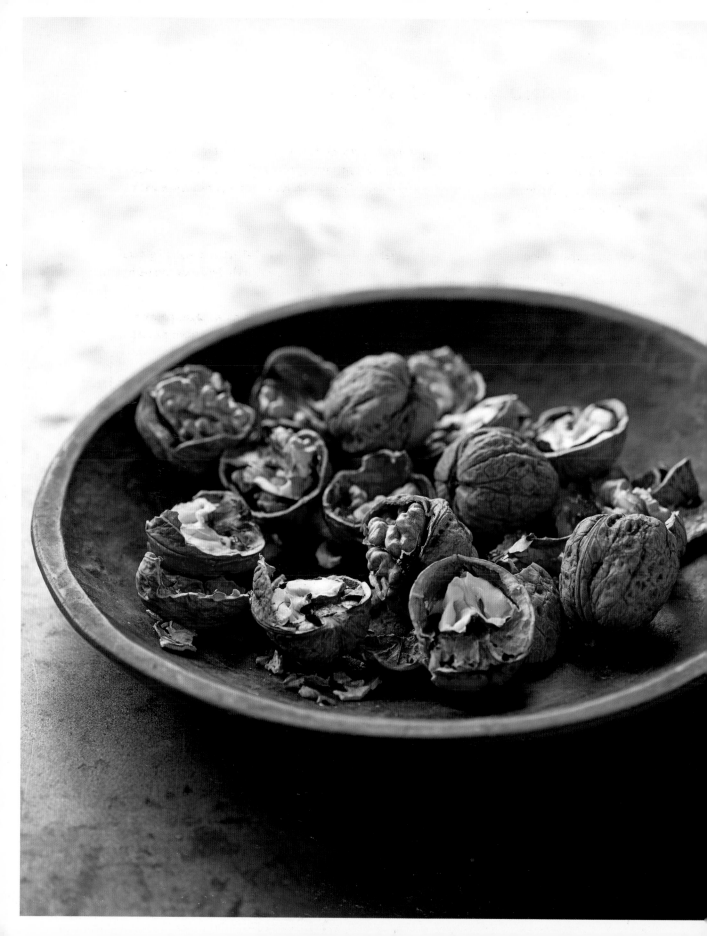

BANANA AND WALNUT BREAD

▲WF ▲GF   MAKES 1 LOAF

This beautiful banana bread, with hints of walnut, nutmeg and cinnamon, will bring a skip to your step and a smile to your dial, and is a fabulous way to enjoy the bountiful health benefits that bananas have to offer, without the risk of mushy messes. Enjoy as an occasional treat warmed with a spread of organic butter.

200 g (7 oz/2 cups) almond meal

60 g (2¼ oz/½ cup) finely chopped walnuts

½ teaspoon gluten-free baking powder

1 teaspoon bicarbonate of soda (baking soda)

½ teaspoon Celtic sea salt

1 teaspoon ground cinnamon

½ teaspoon freshly grated nutmeg

1 teaspoon alcohol-free vanilla extract

8 drops stevia liquid

3 organic eggs

125 g (4½ oz) unsalted butter, melted

60 ml (2 fl oz/¼ cup) additive-free coconut milk

3 ripe bananas, mashed

Preheat the oven to 175°C (345°F/Gas 3–4) and grease and line a 20 x 9 cm (8 x 3½ inch) loaf (bar) tin with baking paper.

Combine the almond meal, walnuts, baking powder, bicarbonate of soda, salt, cinnamon, nutmeg, vanilla and stevia in a bowl and stir to combine.

In a separate bowl, whisk the eggs, butter and coconut milk together. Add to the dry ingredients and fold through. Add the banana and fold in lightly.

Spoon the batter into the prepared tin and bake it in the oven for 30–40 minutes, or until a skewer inserted into the middle of the loaf comes out clean.

Remove from the oven and let it cool in the tin before turning out onto a wire rack.

▶HEALTH BENEFITS◀

If you're feeling a bit sluggish or afflicted in your digestion, bananas are a must-have ingredient to get your system back on track. They will help you absorb and reap the benefits of the foods you are eating. Bananas are excellent for stomach and intestinal inflammations and are a good source of pre-biotics in the form of fructooligosaccharides (FOS), which nourish and feed friendly bacteria in the colon, keeping your intestinal flora and your immune system strong.

INDEX

Page numbers in *italics* refer to photographs.

ACKNOWLEDGEMENTS

I would like to extend a huge thank you to my publisher Murdoch Books in particular Diana Hill, the amazing and wonderful Claire Grady, Miriam Steenhauer and Julia Gregg for your excitement and positivity about this book. Thank you to Steve Brown who did a fantastic job creating gorgeous photos and creative food stylists extraordinaire, Sarah O'Brien and Trish Heagerty.

A massive thanks to all of my recipe testers for happily cooking and tasting the recipes and giving me your feedback and to my amazing researcher Jessica Lowe. To all my friends and colleagues who have been so generous with their time and advice, Grahame Grassby, Louise Cornege, Lise Hearns, Mike Conway, Georgie Bridge, Howard Porter, Meredith Gaston, Holly McBride, Kim Cotton, Alex Swainston Stewart, Marrianne Little, Laura Minford, Juliet Potter, Tom Cronin, Cindy Sciberras and Erica Luiz. Thanks to my family Alex von Kotze, Arizona, Ben, Carol, Clive, Lorraine and Roxy for your love and support. A special huge thanks to the spectacular Cashew Holmes, Justin Smidmore my most favourite person in the world and the incredible Tamsin Rose Holmes who lights up my life.

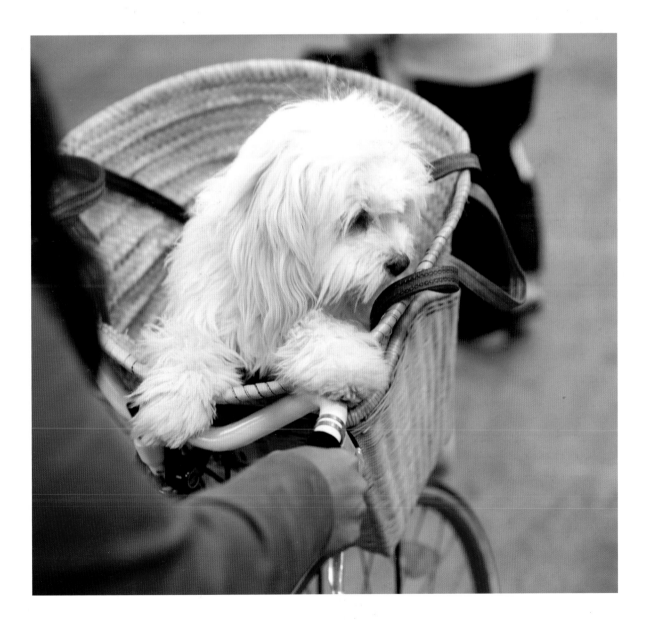

Published in 2014 by Murdoch Books, an imprint of Allen & Unwin.

Murdoch Books Australia
83 Alexander Street
Crows Nest NSW 2065
Phone: +61 (0) 2 8425 0100
Fax: +61 (0) 2 9906 2218
www.murdochbooks.com.au
info@murdochbooks.com.au

Murdoch Books UK
Erico House, 6th Floor
93–99 Upper Richmond Road
Putney, London SW15 2TG
Phone: +44 (0) 20 8785 5995
Fax: +44 (0) 20 8785 5985
www.murdochbooks.co.uk
info@murdochbooks.co.uk

For Corporate Orders & Custom Publishing contact Noel Hammond,
National Business Development Manager, Murdoch Books Australia

Publisher: Diana Hill
Photographer: Steve Brown
Styling: Sarah O'Brien with Trish Heagerty
Designer: Miriam Steenhauer
Editor: Claire Grady
Home Economist: Grace Campbell
Production Manager: Karen Small

A cataloguing-in-publication entry is available from the catalogue of the National
Library of Australia at www.nla.gov.au.

A catalogue record for this book is available from the British Library.

Colour reproduction by Splitting Image, Clayton, Victoria.

Printed by Hang Tai Printing Company Limited, China.

The publisher would like to thank Eveleigh Farmers' Market, Sydney for providing
access to the location for the photo shoot, including the stall holders for allowing
us to shoot their produce. Particular thanks goes to Kurrawong Organics, Julie's
Garden Path and The Fungi.

IMPORTANT: Those who might be at risk from the effects of salmonella poisoning
(the elderly, pregnant women, young children and those suffering from immune
deficiency diseases) should consult their doctor with any concerns about eating
raw eggs.

OVEN GUIDE: You may find cooking times vary depending on the oven you are
using. We have used a fan-forced oven in these recipes. As a general rule, set the
temperature for a conventional oven 20°C (35°F) higher than indicated in the
recipe.

MEASURES GUIDE: We have used 20 ml (4 teaspoon) tablespoon measures.
If you are using a 15 ml (3 teaspoon) tablespoon add an extra teaspoon of the
ingredient for each tablespoon specified.